KETO SLOW COOKER

500 Healthy Recipes You'll Want to Make Everyday.

The Complete Guide to Keto Diet Slow Cooking
for Beginners to Improve Your Health and to Lose Weight!

Cover design by Olivia Rhodes
Interior design by Nigel Barnett

ISBN 9798437737460

Table of contents

Soups and Stews.................................... 95

Introduction

My story has been started long before I knew about the keto diet. It seems to me that I was fat from birth. People and in fact me too had an ambiguous attitude towards this. My parents were awing by me and called me donut, while some peers didn't even want to be friends with me and teased me as fat. At first, I ignored everything. I had tremendous support from my family. They have always been with me and for that, I am very grateful to them. But I was growing up and my body didn't change for the better. At 15, my weight was already over 265 lbs. I couldn't wear the clothes that I liked. I only wore oversized clothes. In the yearbook, all the girls were so beautiful, except me - I was too big! After graduating from school, I got severe depression. I jammed all my sorrows with pizza and cola. And thanks to that, I added about 30 more pounds.

One day I woke up and told myself that this couldn't go on any longer. I will lose weight. I started with a complete medical examination. After that, I went to a dietitian and asked him to credit me with a diet that would work! The doctor said that the keto diet would be perfect for me because even then I started having big health problems.

When I started the keto diet, I didn't expect significant results. But wow! What was my surprise to lose 17 pounds in a month. All I did was follow a diet that BTW was delicious, I didn't feel hungry, and I went to the gym 2 times a week. After following the keto diet for a year, I lost around 85 pounds. Standing on the scales, I couldn't believe my eyes. I was happy! Thanks to the keto diet, I became more confident and believed in myself. Now I am a successful woman, beloved wife, and mother!

Anymore I know for sure that being fat is not a sentence. The most important thing is to find a diet that suits you and strictly follow it. I shared my story and want to help everyone who, like me, suffers from excess weight and all the mental and physical problems associated with it. Everything is in our hands and they should never be omitted! Now I will be your support and guide in this difficult path to the perfect body. I am here with you on the pages of this amazing book. I am sure that you can change your life for the better as well as I did! I believe in you! Good luck!

What to Eat and Avoid on the Keto Diet

Meat and poultry

Actually, it is the primary type of food for the Keto diet. It contains 0% of carbs and is rich in potassium, selenium, zinc, and B vitamins. Grass-fed meat and poultry are the most beneficial. It caused by high omega 3 fats and antioxidants content. Bear in mind that Keto diet is a high-fat diet and high consumption of proteins can cause to harder getting of ketosis.

What to eat	Enjoy occasionally	What to avoid
- chicken	- bacon	- breaded meats
- duck	- ham	- processed meats
- goose	- low-fat meat, such as	
- ground beef	skinless chicken breast	
- lamb	- sausage	
- ostrich		
- partridge		
- pheasant		
- pork		
- quail		
- turkey		
- venison		

Fish and Seafood

Fatty fish as salmon is beneficial for the keto diet. Small fish like sardines, herring, etc. are less in toxins. The best option for a keto diet is wild-caught seafood; it has a higher number of omega 3 fats. Scientifically proved that frequent eating of fish improves mental health.

What to eat	Enjoy occasionally	What to avoid
- catfish	- prawns	- breaded fish
- clams	- salmon	
- cod	- sardines	
- crab	- scallops	
- halibut	- shrimp	
- herring	- snapper	
- lobster	- swordfish	
- mackerel	- tilapia	
- Mahi Mahi	- trout	
- mussels	- tuna	
- oysters		

Grain products

Actually, it is needless to say that all grains are forbidden and can't be eaten if you want to achieve ketosis. Grains contain complex carbohydrates that have a feature to be absorbed slower than simple carbohydrates. For better understanding, if the food has keto-friendly carbs, look at the number of starch and sugar. Their number should be minimum.

What to avoid			
- baked goods	- crackers	- oats	- rice
- bread	- flour	- pasta	- wheat
- cereal	- granola	- pizza	
- corn	- muesli	- popcorn	

Nuts and Seeds

These products are heart-healthy and fiber-rich. Nevertheless, eat nuts and seeds as a snack is a bad idea. As usual, the amount of eaten food can be much more than allowed. Nuts like cashews are very insidious and contain a lot of carbohydrates. Replace them with macadamia or pecan.

What to eat		What to avoid
- almonds	- peanuts	- cashews
- chia seeds	- pecans	- pistachio
- flaxseeds	- pumpkin seeds	- chocolate-covered nuts
- hazelnuts	- walnuts	- nut butter (sweetened)
- nut butter (unsweetened)	- macadamia nuts	

Oils and fats

It is the main component of the keto-friendly sauces and dressings.

Olive oil and coconut oil are highly recommending for everyone who decided to follow the keto diet. They are almost perfect it their fatty acid composition. Avoid artificial trans fats which are poison for our body. This type of fats, as usual, used in French fries, margarine, and crackers.

What to eat		What to avoid	
- avocado oil	- pumpkin seed oil	- grapeseed oil	- peanut oil
- coconut oil	- sesame oil	- canola oil	- soybean oil
- hazelnut oil	- walnut oil	- cottonseed oil	- safflower oil
- olive oil		- hydrogenated oils	- processed
		- margarine	vegetable oils

Vegetables

Keto diet cannot work without vegetables, but their usage should be in moderation. Starchy vegetables such as potatoes, sweet potatoes, etc. are deadly for our body and will not bring anything more than overweight. At the same time, vegetables that are low in carbs, are rich in antioxidants and can protect the body from free radicals that damage our cells.

What to eat		What to avoid	
- asparagus	- mushrooms	- carrots	- pumpkin
- avocado	- olives	- corn	- turnips
- broccoli	- onions	- beets	- yams
- cabbage	- tomatoes	- butternut squash	- yuca
- cauliflower	- peppers	- parsnips	- other starchy
- celery	- spinach	- potatoes (both	vegetables
- cucumber	- zucchini	sweet and regular)	
- eggplant	- other nonstarchy		
- leafy greens	vegetables		
- lettuce			

Berries

If you are looking for how to substitute fruits, this is your godsend. Berries contain up to 12 grams of net carbs per 3.5 ounces serving. They are high in fiber and can maintain the health of your body and fight with diseases. Note consumption of a huge amount of berries can be harmful.

What to eat		What to avoid	
- blackberries	- raspberries	- cherries	- melon
- blueberries	- strawberries	- grapes	- watermelon

Eggs

This is the most wholesome food in the world. Use them everywhere you want! Containing less than one gram of carbohydrates, eggs are a wonderful food for the keto lifestyle. Eating eggs reducing the risk of heart disease and save your eyes health.

Note: free-range eggs are healthier options for the keto diet.

What to eat

- chicken eggs
- duck eggs
- goose eggs
- ostrich eggs
- quail eggs

Dairy

High-fat dairy products are awesome for the keto diet. They are calcium-rich full-fat dairy product is nutritious and can make you full longer. Milk lovers should restrict or even cross out this product from the daily meal plan. It is allowed only 1 tablespoon of milk in your drink per day but doesn't abuse it daily.

What to eat	What to avoid
- butter	- fat-free yogurt
- cheese (soft and hard)	- low-fat cheese
- full-fat yogurt	- milk
- heavy cream	- skim milk
- sour cream	- skim mozzarella
	- sweetened yogurt

Fruits

This type of food is high in carbs that's why they should be limited while keto diet. Besides this, almost all fruits are high in glucose and can enhance blood sugar.

Enjoy occasionally	What to avoid	
- lemons	- apples	- peaches
- pomegranates	- bananas	- pears
- limes	- grapefruits	- pineapple
	- limes	- plums
	- mango	- dried fruits
	- oranges	

Condiments

Condiments can make any type of meal awesome. Even a piece of meat will turn into the masterpiece with them. There are only a few products which are better to avoid; nevertheless, nowadays, you can find keto-friendly substitutors in a supermarket.

One more hot tip: putting hot pepper in your meal will reduce the amount of salt you need and make the taste of the dish more saturated.

What to eat	What to avoid
- herbs and spices	- BBQ sauce
- lemon juice	- hot sauces
- mayonnaise with no added sugar	- ketchup
- salad dressings with no added sugar	- maple syrup
- salt and pepper	- salad dressings with added sugar
- vinegar	- sweet dipping sauces
	- tomato sauce

Beans and legumes

There are no ingredients in this food group that would be healthy for a keto diet. Beans and legumes contain fewer carbs in comparison with root vegetables such as potatoes; nevertheless, this type of carbohydrates fastly adds up.

What to avoid

- black beans	- kidney beans	- navy beans	- pinto beans
- chickpeas	- lentils	- peas	- soybeans

Beverages

A variety of keto drinks may shock you. Probably you know that the best beverage for a keto diet is water. Nevertheless, in order to brighten up a little gray everyday life of keto lovers, the consumption of alcoholic beverages is allowed in moderation. For instance, pure forms of alcohol, such as gin, vodka, or tequila can be drunk once per week. They contain zero amounts of carbs. Avoid all sweetened beverages; they are a priori high carbohydrate.

What to drink	Enjoy occasionally	What to avoid
- almond milk	- dry wine	- alcoholic drinks (sweetened)
- bone broth	- hard liquor	- beer
- coffee (unsweetened)	- vodka	- cider
- flax milk	- other low carb alcoholic drinks	- coffee (sweetened)
- tea (unsweetened)		- fruit juice
- water (still and sparkling)		- soda
		- sports drinks
		- smoothies
		- tea (sweetened)
		- wines (sweet)

Sweets

Cakes and cookies cannot help in losing weight in any diet. As for keto, here everything is strict with this. You should try to avoid sugar and sweeteners in any form. Moreover, sweets negatively affect blood sugar and insulin levels.

Enjoy occasionally	What to avoid	
- erythritol	- artificial sweeteners	- ice cream
- stevia	- buns	- pastries
- sucralose	- candy	- pies
	- cakes	- pudding
	- chocolate	- sugar
	- cookies	- tarts
	- custard	

Others

Fast food and processed food contain a huge amount of stabilizers and harmful carbohydrates. The main rule of the Keto diet is avoiding sugar. 99,9% of such food contains harmful sugars. The existence of which in the body negates the achievement of ketosis.

What to avoid

- fast food
- processed foods

Top 10 Slow Cooker Tips

1. Learn the slow cooker limits.

It is a great mistake to use high settings for cooking all meals. As usual high settings are used for preheating an already cooked meal or for tough meat. If we talk about tender vegetables such as summer squashes or onions – try to avoid long cooking under high pressure. Instead of 12 hours cooking on high, set the slow pressure mode and cook it as a maximum for 6 hours.

2. Use the slow cooker liners. No soaking overnight and scrubbing anymore.

Cleaning the slow cooker is one of the most tedious routines. You can use thousands of kitchen cleansers and sponges to keep the kitchen equipment staying like new or just buy slow cooker liners that will not allow your slow cooker to be dirty. The big bonus of the cooker liners is that they can cut the clean-up time in half. The average price of slow cooker liners is around $8 per set. Leave the spare time for self-care, not for cleaning.

3. Put the dairy products, pasta, and small vegetables in the slow cooker at the last turn or the end of cooking.

Long time cooking for dairy products (milk, cheese, etc.) can cause their curdling or spoiling. Along with them, pasta and vegetables can turn into the mash. We recommend you add all of these ingredients within the last 10 minutes or cook them separately on the stovetop. If the contrary isn't said in the cooking instructions.

4. Cook overnight instead of cooking during the day.

There are two reasons to cook overnight. Firstly, some meals taste better after staying cooked for some time. Such meals are beans, soups, and meat. They get a more tender and succulent flavor.

Secondly, you shouldn't care if your meal is overcooked or cook all in hurry. Come home with the ideas of how to enjoy your evening not with thoughts about overcooked meals.

5. No panic! Too much liquid is not a problem anymore.

Sometimes while using the frozen ingredients you can overestimate the needed amount of liquid. If you are faced with such a problem, just take the excess liquid with the help of the spoon or soup ladle.

6. Feel free to shorten the preparation time.

A slow cooker is a favorite kitchen appliance for a lot because of its simplicity. If your slow cooker recipe provides a long preparation time – just avoid it; most of all meals such as stews, soups, casseroles, etc., implies easy manual – "put all ingredients in the slow cooker bowl and set the desired mode". It doesn't mean you can't use the lifehacks during cooking to emphasize the taste. For instance, browning the meat or frying onion in advance can directly amend the flavor of the final dish and as a result, will increase the preparation time.

7. Cook the cheap cuts of meat.

A slow cooker is a perfect find for cooking cheap cuts of meat such as pork shoulder or chicken thighs. This kitchen equipment has a feature to make saturated palatable meat flavor with fewer meat cuts.

8. Get rid of fat from meat before slow cooking.

The technology of cooking in the slow cooker allows not to add any fat. This is your chance to cook healthier meals without extra effort.

9. Don't throw mashed vegetables – use them as gravy

A lot of recipes suggest adding vegetables while cooking meat meals. At the end of cooking, there is a question: what to do with all remaining mashed vegetables? There is a wonderful trick. You can pull the meat out of the slow cooker bowl and blend all left content with the help of the immersion blender. After this, simmer the mixture for few minutes and voila – it is ready!

10. Make all your favorite recipes slow cooker-friendly

Converting the ordinary recipes into slow cooker recipes is easier than you can think. Follow the rules below:

- If the meal provides 15-30 minutes cooking time, cook it for 1-2-hour on High or 4-6 hours on Low.
- For 30 minutes – 1-hour cooking time, cook the meal for 2-3 hours on High and 5-7 hours on Low.
- The meal that is cooked for 2-4 hours will take 4-6 hours on High and 8-12 hours on low.

Some vegetables, such as root vegetables have longer cooking times. It is recommended to put them at the bottom of the pot and only after this, add all other ingredients.

Top 10 Keto Diet Tips

1. Combine together Keto and Intermittent fasting.

Intermittent fasting (IF) is the right way to get ketosis. It gives your body additional benefits.

Scientists showed that connection keto diet and intermittent fasting can up the results which can give only strict following of the keto diet.

IF means not eating and drinking during a determined amount of time. It is recommended to separate your day into a building phase (BP) and cleansing phase(CP); where the building phase is the time between the first and last time of eating (first-last); and cleansing is the opposite time (last-first). Start from 14-hours CP and 11-hours BP. Continue like this till your body adapts to the new daily plan. It can take 2-3 days. The first days will be the hardest but then you will feel relief and you can safely proceed to the next stage where BP turns into 5 hours and CP - into 19 hours.

According to research, women get the highest benefits of IF. It is possible to get rid of adrenal fatigue, hypothyroid, and hormonal imbalance.

2. Staying hydrated is essential.

Our body is 60% water. Water ensures the normal digestion of food and the absorption of nutrients from the intestines. If there is not enough water in the body, there will be discomfort in the abdomen and constipation. Drinking water is important even if you are not on keto.

The kidneys filter 5,000 ounces of blood per day so that the result is 50 ounces of urine. For the normal elimination of toxins and waste substances, you need to drink at least 50 ounces of water per day, but preferably more.

Many people face the problem of unwillingness to drink water. The best way to prevent dehydration and all its unpleasant consequences is to put a bottle or cup of water on the table and take a sip every time you look at the water. If you realize that you are thirsty, then eliminate thirst in time.

Regular drinking of the right amount of water for 1 week will become a habit and you will not be able to live differently.

3. Salt isn't harmful.

Salt plays an important role in complex metabolic processes. It is part of the blood, lymph, saliva, tears, gastric juice, bile - that is, all the fluids of our body. Any fluctuations in the salt content in the blood plasma lead to serious metabolic disorders

When fewer carbohydrates enter the body, insulin levels drop. Less insulin circulating in the body leads to secrete excess water in the kidneys instead of holding it. It means that salt and other important minerals and electrolytes are washed out of the body.

Replenish salt is possible by eating bone broths, cucumbers, celeriac, salty keto nuts, and seeds.

The best salts for keto diet are 2 types of salt. Pink salt has a more saturated, saltier taste, and contains calcium, magnesium, and potassium. Sea salt is simply evaporated seawater. The crystals of sea salt are slightly larger than iodized salt, and it has a stronger aroma. It contains potassium, magnesium, sulfur, phosphorus, and zinc.

4. Sport is important.

It is proved that physical activity improves the health of the whole body in general and accelerates metabolism. When we do sport, the first thing is we get rid of carbohydrates, and only then we burn fats.

On a keto diet, even minimal physical activity contributes to the rapid decomposition of fats. You simply don't have glucose (carbohydrates) and any load breaks down fats. The most effective workouts on an empty stomach. Sports during keto are very comfortable. You do not feel hungry and can play sports without breakdowns and overeating. Your stamina is significantly increased. If the protein is correctly calculated, you don't lose muscle mass with a calorie deficit.

The combination of three types of workouts gives the best result for health, weight dynamics, and even mood! These are workouts, aerobic, and stretching. Start with small loads every day and increase it as you can. Do not forget to take measurements of your body to monitor the result!

5. Reduce stress.

Sometimes, observing all the postulates of the keto lifestyle, ketosis does not occur or occurs very slowly. In 99 cases, it happens due to the level of stress in your life. Thus, the hormone cortisol rises, the sympathetic nervous system is stimulated.

Cortisol is produced in response to any stress, even the most minor. How does it happen?

Cortisol "eats" our muscles to turn them into glucose, it catabolizes bones, which is fraught with osteoporosis, causes increased appetite, and suppresses immunity. It also causes increased production of glucose and insulin, and exactly this stops ketosis.

During keto-adaptation (the first 3 weeks), increased cortisol is produced, because the usual energy, glucose, ceases to flow into the body, and it turns on the "self-preservation mode".

It is very important at first to minimize stress from the outside, then everything will normalize.

You should be able to switch from stimulation of the sympathetic nervous system to parasympathetic. Stimulation of the parasympathetic nervous system contributes to the restoration and accumulation of energy resources. This can be achieved by a simple 15 minutes' meditation. The time when you cannot be interrupted.

6. Sleep above all!

Sleep and stress are two interconnected components. Lack of sleep leads to increased stress. Consequently, stress hormone levels and blood sugar levels rise and we gain weight very fast.

Doctors recommend an 8-9 hour sleep every day. The best time to fall asleep is before 11 pm. An hour before bedtime, try not to use any gadgets. It is better to spend this time in silence, meditation, listening to calm music or reading a paper book. Thus, we calm the nervous system and set it to sleep. If your stress level per day was high, try to spend more time sleeping. it is the sleep that contributes to our weight loss and getting rid of all diseases. There are some tips to improve your sleep comfort:
- Keep cool in the room. The optimum temperature should not exceed 65-70F.
- Use a black mask for sleeping and earplugs.
- Provide good room ventilation.

7. Don't forget about vegetables.

It is obvious that the main resource of vitamins and minerals is vegetables. You can't cross out them totally from daily meals. Consuming them during the keto diet is very important, but should be in moderation. Starchy vegetables such as sweet potatoes and potatoes are not allowed. Nevertheless, at the same time, you can safely substitute them with broccoli, kale, spinach, white cabbage, Brussels sprouts to your diet. Such vegetables are not only low-carb, but also low-calorie and have a huge number of vitamins, antioxidants, and minerals. They will help you stay full for a long time and protect from eating an extra serving of nuts.

One of the tips of keto coaches is to pamper yourself with low-carb berries once a week. At the same time, it is very important to increase physical activity during this day. Cycling will be just right. All this will fill your body with useful antioxidants and will not add extra pounds.

8. MCT oil is a treasure for a keto diet.

MCT oil is medium-chain triglyceride oil. It practically doesn't require splitting in the small intestine and is absorbed already in the duodenum, going directly to the liver. MCT oil is used by the body as an energy source, which leads to an increase in fat loss. On the other hand, MCT oil isn't deposited in body fat like fatty tissue in comparison with other fatty acids, and it has been shown that it improves thermogenesis, that is, the process during which the body creates heat using excess energy.

MCT oils are good for cooking, especially for baking, frying or grilling. This is due to their high point of "smoke", which means that they are very difficult to oxidize from heat and can withstand high temperatures without losing their original chemical structure at room temperature (losing their useful properties). You can also add MTC oil in keto shakes, coffee, tea, and other keto drinks.

9. Do a kitchen audit

The key to getting ketosis is proper low-carb nutrition. Nevertheless, our brain, knowing that somewhere in the fridge or freezer are a bar of chocolate or a package of vanilla ice cream. So it unconsciously creates situations in which we are obliged to eat them. That's why there are no doubts that one of the best tips is to clean your kitchen and all the shelves from the "seducers". Firstly, write a list of food that is not allowed during the diet, and then one by one throw away everything that is on your list. It may seem too radical right away. But just know that all this will help you completely switch to keto life faster and less stressfully for your body. Also, you can make a list of all you have in the fridge and stick this sheet of paper on the fridge. Doing this you will not eat extra snacks during the day.

10. Keep food near you.

Our life is full of events and sometimes we just don't have time to cook. We have a choice to buy high carbohydrate food in the shop or cook the right food by ourselves. All of this needs extra time. That's why you should always have a "healthy snack" with you. No matter what it is. It can be fat bombs, seeds, or nuts. If you have more time, make the keto salads, or find the keto fruits such as avocado and cook the spreads and dips. But bear in mind, you shouldn't cook much in advance. Their expired date is very short. Follow the rule to purchasing all ingredients for snacks in advance, so that they are always in your fridge. This way you can less likely break your diet and get rid of unnecessary overeating. If you don't know what to cook, use the recipe generator which can help you with the meal for your certain list of food.

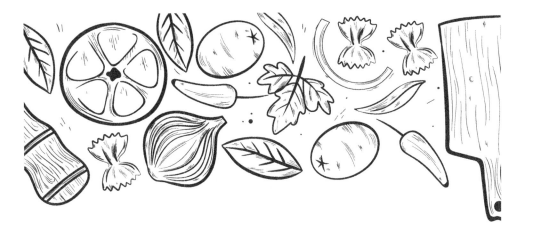

Breakfast

Breakfast Casserole

Yield: 5 servings | **Prep time:** 15 minutes | **Cook time:** 7 hours

Ingredients:
- 1 cup Cheddar cheese, shredded
- 4 oz celery root, chopped
- ½ cup carrot, grated
- 1 teaspoon ground turmeric
- ½ teaspoon cayenne pepper
- 5 eggs, beaten
- ½ cup bell pepper, chopped

Method:
1. Make the layer from celery root in the slow cooker mold.
2. Then put the layer of carrot over the celery root.
3. Sprinkle the vegetables with ground turmeric and cayenne pepper.
4. Then add bell pepper.
5. Pour the beaten eggs over the casserole and top with shredded cheese.
6. Cook the meal on LOW for 7 hours.

Nutritional info per serve: 237 calories, 16.8g protein, 10g carbohydrates, 14.4g fat, 1.7g fiber, 204mg cholesterol, 582mg sodium, 378mg potassium.

Chicken Breakfast Casserole

Prep time: 10 minutes | **Cook time:** 20 minutes | **Yield:** 6 servings

Ingredients:
- 4 chicken fillets, minced
- 1 cup Cheddar cheese, shredded
- ½ cup coconut milk
- 1 teaspoon chili flakes
- 1 teaspoon coconut oil, melted

Method:
1. Preheat the slow cooker on Manual mode for 3 minutes.
2. Then add coconut oil, minced chicken fillet, and chili flakes.
3. Cook the ground chicken on Saute mode for 10 minutes.
4. Then stir it well and add coconut milk and Cheddar cheese.
5. Close the lid and cook the casserole on Manual mode (high pressure) for 10 minutes. Then make a quick pressure release and let the meal cool for 10 minutes.

Nutritional info per serve: 313 calories, 33.3g protein, 1.4g carbohydrates, 19g fat, 0.4g fiber, 106mg cholesterol, 204mg sodium, 308mg potassium.

Egg Casserole

Yield: 4 servings | **Prep time:** 10 minutes | **Cook time:** 2.5 hours

Ingredients:
- 8 oz ham, cut into strips
- 5 eggs, beaten
- 2 tablespoons fresh dill, chopped
- ½ cup heavy cream
- 2 oz Parmesan, grated
- 1 teaspoon ground paprika
- ½ teaspoon avocado oil

Method:
1. Brush the slow cooker with avocado oil from inside.
2. The mix eggs with dill, heavy cream, Parmesan, and ground paprika.
3. After this, put the ham in the bottom of the slow cooker and top with egg mixture.
4. Close and seal the lid.
5. Cook the casserole on High for 2.5 hours.

Nutritional info per serve: 275 calories, 21.6g protein, 4.7g carbohydrates, 19.2g fat, 1.2g fiber, 268mg cholesterol, 957mg sodium, 313mg potassium.

Strawberry Yogurt

Yield: 7 servings | **Prep time:** 15 hours | **Cook time:** 3 hours

Ingredients:
- 4 cup coconut milk
- 1 cup Greek yogurt
- 1 cup strawberries, sliced
- 1 teaspoon coconut shred

Method:
1. Pour the coconut milk into the slow cooker and cook it on HIGH for 3 hours.
2. Cool the coconut milk till it reaches the temperature of 100F.
3. Add Greek yogurt, mix the liquid carefully, and cover with a towel.
4. Leave the yogurt for 10 hours in a warm place.
5. Pour the thick yogurt mixture into the colander or cheese mold and leave for 5 hours to avoid the extra liquid.
6. Transfer the cooked yogurt to the ramekins and top with sliced strawberries and coconut shred.

Nutritional info per serve: 105 calories, 7.6g protein, 9.9g carbohydrates, 4.2g fat, 0.6g fiber, 13mg cholesterol, 76mg sodium, 152mg potassium.

Breakfast Sandwich

Prep time: 10 minutes | **Cook time:** 15 minutes | **Yield:** 4 servings

Ingredients:

- 1 cup lettuce
- 2 cups ground chicken
- 1 tablespoon coconut flour
- 1 teaspoon salt
- 1 tablespoon coconut oil
- ½ teaspoon ground nutmeg
- 3 oz chives, chopped

Method:

1. Preheat the slow cooker on saute mode for 5 minutes.
2. Then add coconut oil and melt it.
3. Add chopped chives.
4. After this, add ground chicken and ground nutmeg. Stir the mixture well and cook for 4 minutes.
5. Then add coconut flour and salt. Sauté the meal for 10 minutes.
6. Fill the lettuce with the ground chicken and transfer it to the plate. The sandwiches are cooked.

Nutritional info per serve: 181 calories, 21.4g protein, 2.6g carbohydrates, 9.2g fat, 1.4g fiber, 62mg cholesterol, 647mg sodium, 254mg potassium.

Zucchini Crumble

Yield: 2 servings | **Prep time:** 10 minutes | **Cook time:** 5 hours

Ingredients:

- 1 tablespoon Erythritol
- 1 zucchini, roughly grated
- 4 oz chia seeds
- 4 tablespoons water
- 1 tablespoon almond butter
- 1 teaspoon vanilla extract

Method:

1. Put the zucchini in the slow cooker.
2. Add water, almond butter, vanilla extract, and Erythritol.
3. Cook the zucchini for 5 hours on Low.
4. Then stir them carefully.
5. Put the cooked zucchinis and chia seeds one-by-one in the serving glasses.

Nutritional info per serve: 208 calories, 7.6g protein, 20.5g carbohydrates, 13.4g fat, 11.6g fiber, 0mg cholesterol, 16mg sodium, 435mg potassium.

Frittata with Greens

Prep time: 10 minutes | **Cook time:** 10 minutes | **Yield:** 2 servings

Ingredients:

- 2 eggs, beaten
- ¼ cup heavy cream
- ½ teaspoon white pepper
- 1 tablespoon chives, chopped
- 1 teaspoon ground paprika
- 1 teaspoon butter, softened
- 1 tablespoon scallions, chopped
- 1 cup water, for cooking

Method:

1. In the mixing bowl, mix eggs with heavy cream, white pepper, chives, ground paprika, and scallions.
2. Then grease the frittata mold with softened butter.
3. Pour the egg mixture into the prepared ramekin and place it on the trivet.
4. Then pour water into the slow cooker and insert the trivet inside.
5. Cook the frittata for 10 minutes on Manual mode (high pressure).
6. Then make a quick pressure release and cut the meal into halves.

Nutritional info per serve: 137 calories, 6.2g protein, 2g carbohydrates, 12g fat, 0.7g fiber, 189mg cholesterol, 86mg sodium, 116mg potassium.

Coconut Milk Broccoli Rice

Yield: 4 servings | **Prep time:** 10 minutes | **Cook time:** 2 hours

Ingredients:

- 1 cup broccoli rice
- 1 cup of water
- 1 cup coconut milk
- 1 tablespoon Erythritol
- 1 teaspoon vanilla extract
- 1 tablespoon coconut oil
- ¼ teaspoon ground cinnamon

Method:

1. Put all ingredients in the slow cooker and mix.
2. Close the lid and cook the meal on High for 2 hours.
3. Then stir the cooked broccoli rice and transfer it to the serving bowls.

Nutritional info per serve: 178 calories, 2g protein, 8.8g carbohydrates, 17.8g fat, 2g fiber, 0mg cholesterol, 18mg sodium, 233mg potassium.

Egg Cups

Prep time: 15 minutes | **Cook time:** 13 minutes | **Yield:** 4 servings

Ingredients:
- 4 eggs
- ¼ cups spinach, chopped
- ½ teaspoon chili flakes
- 2 oz Mozzarella, sliced
- 1 teaspoon butter, melted
- 1 cup water, for cooking

Method:
1. Brush the muffin molds with melted butter.
2. Then crack the egg in every mold and sprinkle them with chili flakes and chopped spinach.
3. Top the eggs with sliced Mozzarella.
4. Pour water and insert the steamer rack into the slow cooker.
5. Put the egg cups on the rack and close the lid.
6. Cook the meal on manual mode (high pressure) for 3 minutes. Make a quick pressure release.
7. Let the cooked egg cups cool to room temperature. Remove the eggs from the muffin molds.

Nutritional info per serve: 112 calories, 9.6g protein, 0.9g carbohydrates, 7.8g fat, 0g fiber, 174mg cholesterol, 155mg sodium, 70mg potassium.

Zucchini and Broccoli Mix

Yield: 3 servings | **Prep time:** 10 minutes | **Cook time:** 3 hours

Ingredients:
- ½ zucchini, grated
- 1 teaspoon coconut oil
- 1 cup broccoli rice
- 2 cup chicken stock
- 1 tablespoon cream cheese
- 1 oz goat cheese, crumbled

Method:
1. Mix grated zucchini with coconut oil, broccoli rice, and chicken stock and transfer to the slow cooker.
2. Then add cream cheese.
3. Cook the meal on High for 3 hours.
4. Then stir the cooked broccoli rice well and transfer to the serving plates.
5. Top the meal with crumbled goat cheese.

Nutritional info per serve: 67 calories, 3.6g protein, 2.9g carbohydrates, 4.9g fat, 0.9g fiber, 10mg cholesterol, 424mg sodium, 150mg potassium.

Bacon and Cheese Bites

Prep time: 15 minutes | **Cook time:** 3 minutes | **Yield:** 2 servings

Ingredients:
- 2 tablespoons coconut flour
- ½ cup Cheddar cheese, shredded
- 2 teaspoons coconut milk
- 2 bacon slices, cooked
- ½ teaspoon dried parsley
- 1 cup water, for cooking

Method:
1. In the mixing bowl, mix up coconut flour, Cheddar cheese, coconut milk, and dried parsley.
2. Then chop the cooked bacon and add it to the mixture. Mix the ingredients
3. Pour water and insert the trivet in the slow cooker.
4. Line the trivet with baking paper. After this, make the small balls (bites) from the cheese mixture and put them on the prepared trivet.
5. Cook the meal for 3 minutes on manual mode (high pressure).
6. Then make a quick pressure release and cool the cooked meal well.

Nutritional info per serve: 288 calories, 16.2g protein, 8.9g carbohydrates, 20.5g fat, 5.1g fiber, 51mg cholesterol, 645mg sodium, 150mg potassium.

Chocolate Toast

Yield: 4 servings | **Prep time:** 10 minutes | **Cook time:** 20 minutes

Ingredients:
- 4 keto cloud bread
- 1 tablespoon vanilla extract
- 1 oz dark chocolate, chopped
- 1 tablespoon coconut oil
- ¼ cup heavy cream

Method:
1. Mix vanilla extract, chocolate, coconut oil, and heavy cream.
2. Pour the mixture into the slow cooker and cook on High for 20 minutes.
3. Make a quick pressure release and stir the mixture, cool it.
4. Spread the cloud bread with a cooked mixture.

Nutritional info per serve: 102 calories, 0.7g protein, 4.8g carbohydrates, 8.3g fat, 0.2g fiber, 12mg cholesterol, 9mg sodium, 37mg potassium.

Chocolate Keto Rice

Yield: 5 servings | **Prep time:** 10 minutes | **Cook time:** 4 hours

Ingredients:
- 1 oz dark chocolate, chopped
- 1 teaspoon vanilla extract
- 2 cups of coconut
- milk
- 1 cup broccoli rice
- ½ teaspoon ground cardamom

Method:
1. Put all ingredients in the slow cooker and stir carefully with the help of the spoon.
2. Close the lid and cook the meal for 4 hours on Low.

Nutritional info per serve: 379 calories, 7.5g protein, 3g carbohydrates, 27.2g fat, 6.1g fiber, 1mg cholesterol, 19mg sodium, 374mg potassium.

Cheese Baked Eggs

Prep time: 15 minutes | **Cook time:** 30 minutes | **Yield:** 4 servings

Ingredients:
- 4 eggs
- ½ cup Mozzarella, shredded
- 1 tablespoon coconut oil, melted
- ½ teaspoon chili powder

Method:
1. Grease the ramekins with coconut oil.
2. Then crack the eggs inside.
3. Add chili powder and Mozzarella.
4. Place the ramekins in the slow cooker and cook the meal on High for 30 minutes.

Nutritional info per serve: 103 calories, 6.6g protein, 0.7g carbohydrates, 8.5g fat, 0.1g fiber, 166mg cholesterol, 86mg sodium, 65mg potassium.

Butternut Squash Pate

Yield: 7 servings | **Prep time:** 7 minutes | **Cook time:** 4 hours

Ingredients:
- 8 oz butternut squash puree
- 1 tablespoon Erythritol
- 1 teaspoon cinnamon
- ¼ teaspoon ground
- clove
- 1 tablespoon lemon juice
- 2 tablespoons coconut oil

Method:
1. Put all ingredients in the slow cooker, gently stir, and cook on Low for 4 hours.

Nutritional info per serve: 63 calories, 0g protein, 6.9g carbohydrates, 3.9g fat, 0.8g fiber, 0mg cholesterol, 3mg sodium, 7mg potassium.

Creamy Broccoli with Pecan

Yield: 7 servings | **Prep time:** 10 minutes | **Cook time:** 3 hours

Ingredients:
- 1 oz pecans, crushed
- 2 cups broccoli rice
- 1 cup heavy cream
- 1 cup of water
- ¼ teaspoon chili flakes
- 1 oz Parmesan, grated

Method:
1. Put broccoli rice, heavy cream, water, and chili flakes in the slow cooker.
2. Cook the ingredients on High for 3 hours.
3. Then add grated cheese and crushed pecans.
4. Stir the meal well and transfer to the serving plates.

Nutritional info per serve: 109 calories, 2.8g protein, 2.9g carbohydrates, 10.2g fat, 1.1g fiber, 2.6mg cholesterol, 54mg sodium, 112mg potassium.

Bacon Casserole

Prep time: 10 minutes | **Cook time:** 10 minutes | **Yield:** 6 servings

Ingredients:
- 4 bacon slices, chopped
- 1 teaspoon avocado oil
- 6 eggs, beaten
- ½ cup spinach, chopped
- ½ cup organic almond milk
- 1 teaspoon chili flakes
- 3 oz Cheddar cheese, shredded
- 1 cup water, for cooking

Method:
1. Preheat the slow cooker on Saute mode for 2-3 minutes.
2. Then put the chopped bacon inside and cook it on saute mode for 5 minutes or until it is crunchy.
3. Then transfer the cooked bacon to the mixing bowl. Add the eggs, spinach, almond milk, chili flakes, and Cheddar cheese. Carefully stir the. Clean the slow cooker and pour water and insert the steamer rack inside.
4. After this, pour the mixture into the baking mold/ramekin and cover it with foil. Cook the casserole on manual (high pressure) for 15 minutes. Allow the natural pressure release for 10 minutes.

Nutritional info per serve: 236 calories, 14.3g protein, 2g carbohydrates, 19.2g fat, 0.5g fiber, 193mg cholesterol, 447mg sodium, 214mg potassium.

Morning Pie

Yield: 6 servings | **Prep time:** 10 minutes | **Cook time:** 3 hours

Ingredients:

- ½ cup broccoli rice
- 1 cups heavy cream
- 1 cup butternut squash, diced
- 1 teaspoon vanilla extract
- ½ teaspoon ground cinnamon
- 1 teaspoon avocado oil
- 4 pecans, crushed

Method:

1. Mix broccoli rice and heavy cream in the slow cooker.
2. Add diced butternut squash, vanilla extract, and ground cinnamon.
3. Then add avocado oil and pecans.
4. Carefully mix the ingredients and close the lid.
5. Cook the pie on Low for 3 hours.
6. Then cool the pie and cut it into servings.

Nutritional info per serve: 151 calories, 1.9g protein, 5.4g carbohydrates, 14.2g fat, 1.8g fiber, 27mg cholesterol, 11mg sodium, 164mg potassium.

Homemade Starbucks Eggs

Prep time: 10 minutes | **Cook time:** 2 minutes | **Yield:** 2 servings

Ingredients:

- 4 eggs
- 2 oz cream cheese
- 1/3 cup Cheddar cheese, shredded
- 1 teaspoon chives, chopped
- 1 cup of water

Method:

1. Crack the eggs in the bowl and mix them with chives.
2. Whisk the eggs and add shredded Cheddar cheese and cream cheese. Stir well.
3. Then pour the eggs into the muffin molds.
4. Pour water into the slow cooker and insert the steamer rack.
5. Place the eggs on the rack and cook them for 2 minutes on Manual mode (high pressure).
6. Make a quick pressure release and remove the eggs from the molds.

Nutritional info per serve: 301 calories, 17.9g protein, 1.7g carbohydrates, 24.9g fat, 0g fiber, 378mg cholesterol, 328mg sodium, 173mg potassium.

Egg Sandwich

Yield: 4 servings | **Prep time:** 10 minutes | **Cook time:** 2.5 hours

Ingredients:

- 4 keto cloud bread
- 4 eggs, beaten
- 4 ham slices
- 1 teaspoon smoked paprika
- ½ teaspoon ground turmeric
- ½ teaspoon minced garlic
- 1 tablespoon coconut oil

Method:

1. In the bowl mix eggs, smoked paprika, ground turmeric, and minced garlic.
2. Then dip every cloud bread in the egg mixture.
3. Put the coconut oil in the slow cooker.
4. Arrange the cloud bread slices in the slow cooker in one layer and top with ham.
5. Close the lid and cook the meal on HIGH for 2.5 hours.

Nutritional info per serve: 165 calories, 11g protein, 6.6g carbohydrates, 10.6g fat, 0.9g fiber, 180mg cholesterol, 488mg sodium, 169mg potassium.

Stuffed Hard-Boiled Eggs

Prep time: 10 minutes | **Cook time:** 5 minutes | **Yield:** 6 servings

Ingredients:

- 6 eggs
- 3 oz Provolone cheese, grated
- 1 teaspoon chili pepper, chopped
- 1 tablespoon organic almond milk
- ½ teaspoon ground paprika
- 1 cup of water

Method:

1. Pour water into the slow cooker.
2. Add eggs and close the lid.
3. Cook the on manual mode (high pressure) for 5 minutes. Then allow the natural pressure release and open the lid.
4. Cool and peel the eggs.
5. After this, cut the eggs into halves and remove the egg yolks.
6. Mash the egg yolks and mix them up with grated cheese, almond milk, chili pepper, and ground paprika.
7. Then fill the egg white halves with an egg yolk mixture.

Nutritional info per serve: 119 calories, 9.3g protein, 1g carbohydrates, 8.8g fat, 0.2g fiber, 173mg cholesterol, 186mg sodium, 92mg potassium.

White Cabbage Hash Browns

Prep time: 10 minutes | **Cook time:** 10 minutes | **Yield:** 3 servings

Ingredients:

- 1 cup white cabbage, shredded
- 3 eggs, beaten
- ½ teaspoon ground nutmeg
- 1 tablespoon avocado oil
- ½ teaspoon onion powder
- ½ zucchini, grated

Method:

1. In the mixing bowl, mix up shredded cabbage, eggs, ground nutmeg, onion powder, and grated zucchini.
2. Then heat avocado oil in the slow cooker on Saute mode.
3. Make the medium hash browns from the cabbage mixture (use the tablespoon for this step).
4. After this, place the hash browns in the hot avocado oil.
5. Cook them on saute mode for 4 minutes from each side.

Nutritional info per serve: 84 calories, 6.4g protein, 3.5g carbohydrates, 2.2g fat, 1.2g fiber, 164mg cholesterol, 70mg sodium, 204mg potassium.

Broccoli Quiche

Yield: 8 servings | **Prep time:** 10 minutes | **Cook time:** 5 hours

Ingredients:

- 2 tablespoons broccoli rice
- 1 cup broccoli, chopped
- ½ cup fresh cilantro, chopped
- ¼ cup Mozzarella, shredded
- 1 teaspoon olive oil
- 8 eggs, beaten
- 1 teaspoon ground paprika

Method:

1. Brush the slow cooker bowl with olive oil.
2. In the mixing bowl mix broccoli rice, eggs, and ground paprika.
3. Pour the mixture into the slow cooker.
4. Add all remaining ingredients, gently stir the mixture.
5. Close the lid and cook the quiche for 5 hours on High.

Nutritional info per serve: 80 calories, 6.3g protein, 2.2g carbohydrates, 5.3g fat, 0.6g fiber, 164mg cholesterol, 71mg sodium, 111mg potassium.

Swedish Meatballs

Prep time: 15 minutes | **Cook time:** 25 minutes | **Yield:** 2 servings

Ingredients:

- 1/3 cup ground beef
- ¼ cup ground pork
- ¼ teaspoon ground black pepper
- 1 teaspoon coconut oil, melted
- 1 teaspoon almond flour
- ¼ teaspoon Erythritol
- ½ cup organic almond milk

Method:

1. In the mixing bowl, mix up ground beef, ground pork, ground black pepper, and Erythritol.
2. Make the small meatballs.
3. Preheat the slow cooker on saute mode for 2 minutes and add melted coconut oil.
4. Put the meatballs in the hot oil in one layer and cook them for 3 minutes from each side.
5. Meanwhile, mix up almond milk and coconut flour.
6. Pour the liquid over the meatballs and close the lid. Cook the meal on saute mode for 15 minutes.

Nutritional info per serve: 276 calories, 17.1g protein, 3.8g carbohydrates, 21.7g fat, 1.6g fiber, 49mg cholesterol, 136mg sodium, 240mg potassium.

Spinach Frittata

Yield: 6 servings | **Prep time:** 10 minutes | **Cook time:** 2 hours

Ingredients:

- 2 cups spinach, chopped
- 1 teaspoon smoked paprika
- 1 teaspoon avocado
- oil
- 7 eggs, beaten
- 2 tablespoons coconut oil
- ¼ cup heavy cream

Method:

1. Mix eggs with heavy cream.
2. Then grease the slow cooker with coconut oil and pour the egg mixture inside.
3. Add smoked paprika, sesame oil, and spinach.
4. Carefully mix the ingredients and close the lid.
5. Cook the frittata on High for 2 hours.

Nutritional info per serve: 140 calories, 6.9g protein, 1.1g carbohydrates, 12.3g fat, 0.4g fiber, 198mg cholesterol, 82mg sodium, 137mg potassium.

Romano Cheese Frittata

Yield: 4 servings | **Prep time:** 10 minutes | **Cook time:** 3 hours

Ingredients:
- 4 oz Romano cheese, grated
- 5 eggs, beaten
- ¼ cup of coconut milk
- ½ cup bell pepper, chopped
- ½ teaspoon ground white pepper
- 1 teaspoon olive oil
- ½ teaspoon ground coriander

Method:
1. Mix eggs with coconut milk, ground white pepper, bell pepper, and ground coriander.
2. Then brush the slow cooker bowl with olive oil.
3. Pour the egg mixture into the slow cooker.
4. Cook the frittata on High for 2.5 hours.
5. Then top the frittata with Romano cheese and cook for 30 minutes on High.

Nutritional info per serve: 238 calories, 16.5g protein, 3.6g carbohydrates, 17.9g fat, 0.6g fiber, 234mg cholesterol, 420mg sodium, 169mg potassium.

Bell Peppers with Omelet

Prep time: 10 minutes | **Cook time:** 30 minutes | **Yield:** 2 servings

Ingredients:
- 1 large bell pepper, trimmed
- 2 eggs, beaten
- 1 tablespoon coconut milk
- ¼ teaspoon dried oregano
- 1 cup of water

Method:
1. Cut the bell peppers into halves and remove the seeds.
2. After this, in the mixing bowl mix up eggs, coconut milk, and oregano.
3. Pour water into the slow cooker and insert the rack.
4. Then pour the egg mixture into the pepper halves.
5. Transfer the peppers to the rack and close the lid.
6. Cook the meal on Manual mode (high pressure) for 30 minutes. Then make a quick pressure release.

Nutritional info per serve: 100 calories, 6.3g protein, 5.4g carbohydrates, 6.3g fat, 1.1g fiber, 164mg cholesterol, 68mg sodium, 195mg potassium.

Meat and Cauliflower Bake

Prep time: 10 minutes | **Cook time:** 15 minutes | **Yield:** 4 servings

Ingredients:
- 4 eggs, beaten
- 1 cup cauliflower, shredded
- ½ cup ground chicken
- 1 tablespoon Italian seasonings
- ¼ cup Cheddar cheese, shredded
- 1 cup water, for cooking

Method:
1. In the mixing bowl, mix up beaten eggs, shredded cauliflower, and Italian seasonings.
2. Then pour the mixture into 4 ramekins.
3. Add ground chicken.
4. Top the ramekins with Cheddar cheese.
5. Then pour the water into the slow cooker, insert the trivet.
6. Put the ramekins on the trivet and close the lid.
7. Cook the meal on manual mode (high pressure) for 15 minutes. Then make a quick pressure release.

Nutritional info per serve: 142 calories, 12.9g protein, 2.1g carbohydrates, 9.1g fat, 0.6g fiber, 189mg cholesterol, 129mg sodium, 186mg potassium.

Sausage Frittata

Yield: 5 servings | **Prep time:** 10 minutes | **Cook time:** 4 hours

Ingredients:
- ½ onion, diced
- 8 oz sausages, handmade, chopped
- 1 teaspoon olive oil
- 1 cup Mozzarella, shredded
- 6 eggs, beaten
- ½ teaspoon cayenne pepper

Method:
1. Put sausages in the slow cooker.
2. Add onion and coconut oil.
3. Close the lid and cook the ingredients on high for 2 hours.
4. Then stir them well.
5. Add eggs, cayenne pepper, and shredded mozzarella.
6. Carefully stir the meal and close the lid.
7. Cook it on high for 2 hours.

Nutritional info per serve: 258 calories, 17.2g protein, 1.7g carbohydrates, 20.1g fat, 0.3g fiber, 238mg cholesterol, 448mg sodium, 224mg potassium.

Butter Broccoli

Yield: 4 serving | **Prep time:** 5 minutes | **Cook time:** 10 minutes

Ingredients:

- 1 tablespoon Erythritol
- 1 tablespoon coconut shred
- 1 teaspoon vanilla extract
- 1 cup of water
- ½ cup heavy cream
- 1 cup broccoli rice
- 2 tablespoons butter

Method:

1. Put butter, broccoli rice, heavy cream, water, vanilla extract, and coconut shred in the slow cooker.
2. Carefully stir the ingredients and close the lid.
3. Cook the meal on Low for 5 hours.
4. Then add Erythritol, stir it, and transfer it to the serving bowls.

Nutritional info per serve: 212 calories, 3.1g protein, 19.2g carbohydrates, 13.9g fat, 2.3g fiber, 36mg cholesterol, 51mg sodium, 92mg potassium.

Broccoli Omelet

Yield: 4 servings | **Prep time:** 10 minutes | **Cook time:** 2 hours

Ingredients:

- 5 eggs, beaten
- 1 tablespoon cream cheese
- 3 oz broccoli, chopped
- 1 tomato, chopped
- 1 teaspoon avocado oil

Method:

1. Mix eggs with cream cheese and transfer in the slow cooker.
2. Add avocado oil, broccoli, and tomato.
3. Close the lid and cook the omelet on High for 2 hours.

Nutritional info per serve: 99 calories, 7.9g protein, 2.6g carbohydrates, 6.6g fat, 0.8g fiber, 207mg cholesterol, 92mg sodium, 184mg potassium.

Mozzarella Casserole

Yield: 6 servings | **Prep time:** 10 minutes | **Cook time:** 8 hours

Ingredients:

- 1 chili pepper, chopped
- 1 tomato, chopped
- 1 cup Mozzarella, shredded
- 2 tablespoons cream cheese
- 5 oz ham, chopped
- 1 teaspoon garlic powder
- 2 eggs, beaten

Method:

1. Mix chili pepper, tomato, and ham.
2. Add minced garlic and stir the ingredients.
3. Transfer it to the slow cooker and flatten gently.
4. Top the casserole with eggs, cream cheese, and Mozzarella.
5. Cook the casserole on LOW for 8 hours.

Nutritional info per serve: 110 calories, 8.3g protein, 7.2g carbohydrates, 5.8g fat, 1g fiber, 74mg cholesterol, 449mg sodium, 159mg potassium.

Cream Grits

Yield: 2 servings | **Prep time:** 10 minutes | **Cook time:** 5 hours

Ingredients:

- ½ cup keto grits
- ½ cup heavy cream
- 1 cup of water
- 1 tablespoon cream cheese

Method:

1. Put keto grits, heavy cream, and water in the slow cooker.
2. Cook the meal on LOW for 5 hours.
3. When the grits are cooked, add cream cheese and stir carefully.
4. Transfer the meal to the serving bowls.

Nutritional info per serve: 151 calories, 1.6g protein, 6.9g carbohydrates, 13.2g fat, 1g fiber, 47mg cholesterol, 116mg sodium, 33mg potassium.

Coconut Milk Pudding

Yield: 3 servings | **Prep time:** 10 minutes | **Cook time:** 7 hours

Ingredients:

- 1 cup coconut milk
- 3 eggs, beaten
- 2 tablespoons almond flour
- 1 teaspoon vanilla extract
- 1 tablespoon Erythritol

Method:

1. Mix coconut milk with eggs and almond flour.
2. Whisk the mixture until smooth and add vanilla extract and Erythritol.
3. Pour the liquid into the slow cooker and close the lid.
4. Cook the mixture on Low for 7 hours.

Nutritional info per serve: 264 calories, 7.9g protein, 10.4g carbohydrates, 25.7g fat, 2.3g fiber, 12mg cholesterol, 75mg sodium, 271mg potassium.

Poppy Seeds Buns

Yield: 8 servings | **Prep time:** 20 minutes | **Cook time:** 5 hours

Ingredients:

- 3 tablespoon poppy seeds
- 1 egg, beaten
- 6 oz plain cottage cheese
- 1 cup almond flour
- 1 teaspoon ground cardamom
- 2 tablespoons olive oil

Method:

1. Mix poppy seeds with egg, cottage cheese, flour, and ground cardamom.
2. Knead the homogenous dough.
3. Add olive oil and keep kneading the dough for 4 minutes more.
4. After this, make the small buns from the dough and put them in the slow cooker bowl.
5. Close the lid and cook them on High for 5 hours.

Nutritional info per serve: 97 calories, 4.7g protein, 2.3g carbohydrates, 8.2g fat, 0.8g fiber, 49mg cholesterol, 77mg sodium, 33mg potassium.

Bacon Rutabaga

Yield: 4 servings | **Prep time:** 10 minutes | **Cook time:** 5 hours

Ingredients:

- 4 rutabagas, peeled
- 1 teaspoon dried thyme
- 4 teaspoons olive oil
- 4 bacon slices

Method:

1. Cut the rutabagas into halves and sprinkle with dried thyme and olive oil.
2. After this, cut every bacon slice into halves.
3. Put the rutabaga halves in the slow cooker bowl and top with bacon slices.
4. Close the lid and cook them for 5 hours on High.

Nutritional info per serve: 282 calories, 11.7g protein, 18.6g carbohydrates, 13.4g fat, 9.7g fiber, 21mg cholesterol, 452mg sodium, 976mg potassium.

Morning Keto Muesli

Yield: 6 servings | **Prep time:** 10 minutes | **Cook time:** 4 hours

Ingredients:

- 1 cup broccoli rice
- 1 teaspoon chia seeds
- 1 teaspoon sesame seeds
- 1 teaspoon ground cinnamon
- 2 cups of coconut milk

Method:

1. Mix coconut milk with broccoli rice, sesame seeds, and ground cinnamon.
2. Transfer the ingredients to the slow cooker and cook on Low for 4 hours.
3. Then stir carefully and transfer in the serving bowls.

Nutritional info per serve: 199 calories, 2.6g protein, 6.5g carbohydrates, 19.8g fat, 2.9g fiber, 0mg cholesterol, 17mg sodium, 262mg potassium.

Keto Giant Pancake

Yield: 4 servings | **Prep time:** 10 minutes | **Cook time:** 4 hours

Ingredients:

- 1 cup almond flour
- ½ cup coconut milk
- 2 eggs, beaten
- 1 tablespoon coconut oil, melted

Method:

1. Mic almond flour with coconut milk and eggs. Stir the mixture until smooth.
2. Then brush the slow cooker mold with coconut oil from inside.
3. Pour the pancake mixture into the slow cooker and close the lid.
4. Cook it on High for 4 hours.

Nutritional info per serve: 170 calories, 5g protein, 3.3g carbohydrates, 16.2g fat, 1.4g fiber, 82mg cholesterol, 38mg sodium, 108mg potassium.

Asparagus Eggs

Prep time: 10 minutes | **Cook time:** 20 minutes | **Yield:** 2 servings

Ingredients:

- 3 oz asparagus, chopped, boiled
- 4 eggs, beaten
- 1 tablespoon coconut oil, melted

Method:

1. Pour the coconut oil into the slow cooker bowl and preheat for 2 minutes on Saute mode.
2. Add chopped asparagus and eggs.
3. Close the lid and cook the eggs in High-pressure mode for 20 minutes.

Nutritional info per serve: 193 calories, 12g protein, 2.3g carbohydrates, 15.6g fat, 0.9g fiber, 327mg cholesterol, 124mg sodium, 204mg potassium.

Noatmeal

Prep time: 10 minutes | **Cook time:** 5 hours | **Yield:** 4 servings

Ingredients:
- ½ cup coconut shred
- 1 teaspoon ground cinnamon
- 1 teaspoon Erythritol
- 3 tablespoons flaxseeds
- 3 tablespoons sunflower seeds
- ½ cup coconut milk
- ½ cup of water
- ½ teaspoon coconut oil

Method:
1. In the mixing bowl, mix up coconut shred, ground cinnamon, Erythritol, flaxseeds, sunflower seeds, coconut milk, water, and coconut oil.
2. Transfer the mixture to the slow cooker bowl.
3. Set the slow cook mode Porridge and cook the meal for 5 hours on Low.
4. Then stir it well and transfer in the serving ramekins.

Nutritional info per serve: 216 calories, 2.1g protein, 9.3g carbohydrates, 20.5g fat, 4.6g fiber, 0mg cholesterol, 12mg sodium, 138mg potassium.

Morning Burritos

Prep time: 10 minutes | **Cook time:** 15 minutes | **Yield:** 4 servings

Ingredients:
- 4 keto tortillas
- 1 cup ground beef
- ¼ cup crushed tomatoes
- 1 teaspoon coconut oil, melted
- 3 oz chives, chopped
- ½ teaspoon dried cilantro

Method:
1. In the mixing bowl mix up ground beef, crushed tomatoes, coconut oil, chives, and dried cilantro.
2. Put the meat mixture in the slow cooker.
3. Close and seal the lid.
4. Cook the beef mixture for 15 minutes on Manual mode (high pressure).
5. Then make a quick pressure release and stir the meat well.
6. Fill the tortillas with the cooked mixture and roll them in the shape of burritos.

Nutritional info per serve: 237 calories, 19.6g protein, 10.2g carbohydrates, 13.4g fat, 5g fiber, 22mg cholesterol, 294mg sodium, 146mg potassium.

Giant Vanilla Pancake

Prep time: 15 minutes | **Cook time:** 4 hours | **Yield:** 6 servings

Ingredients:
- ½ cup coconut flour
- 3 tablespoons Erythritol
- ¼ cup coconut milk
- 3 eggs, beaten
- 1 teaspoon vanilla extract
- ¼ cup almond flour
- 1 teaspoon baking powder
- Cooking spray

Method:
1. In the mixing bowl, mix up coconut flour, Erythritol, coconut milk, eggs, vanilla extract, and almond flour.
2. Then add baking powder and whisk the mixture until smooth.
3. Pour the pancake mixture into the slow cooker.
4. Cook the meal on manual mode (low pressure) for 4 hours.

Nutritional info per serve: 111 calories, 5.3g protein, 12g carbohydrates, 4.2g fat, 4.4g fiber, 82mg cholesterol, 54mg sodium, 141mg potassium.

Meat Cups

Prep time: 15 minutes | **Cook time:** 30 minutes | **Yield:** 4 servings

Ingredients:
- 4 quill eggs
- 10 oz ground pork
- 1 jalapeno pepper, chopped
- 1 teaspoon dried dill
- 1 tablespoon coconut oil, melted
- 1 cup water, for cooking

Method:
1. In the mixing bowl, mix up ground pork, chopped jalapeno pepper, dill, and coconut oil
2. When the meat mixture is homogenous, transfer it to the silicone muffin molds and press the surface gently.
3. Then pour water into the slow cooker and insert the trivet.
4. Place the meat cups on the trivet.
5. Then crack the eggs over the meat mixture and close the lid.
6. Cook the meal on manual mode (high pressure) for 30 minutes.
7. Then make a quick pressure release.

Nutritional info per serve: 168 calories, 21.8g protein, 0.5g carbohydrates, 8.3g fat, 0.1g fiber, 145mg cholesterol, 76mg sodium, 349mg potassium.

Bacon Avocado Bomb

Prep time: 10 minutes | **Cook time:** 25 minutes | **Yield:** 4 servings

Ingredients:

- 1 avocado, pilled, pitted, halved
- 4 bacon slices
- ½ teaspoon ground cinnamon
- 1 teaspoon coconut milk
- ½ teaspoon chili flakes

Method:

1. Sprinkle the avocado with ground cinnamon and chili flakes.
2. Then fill it with coconut milk and wrap it in the bacon slices.
3. Secure the avocado bomb with toothpicks, if needed, and wrap it in the foil.
4. Place it in the slow cooker and close the lid.
5. Cook the bomb on saute mode for 25 minutes.
6. Then remove the foil and slice the avocado bomb into the servings.

Nutritional info per serve: 209 calories, 8g protein, 4.9g carbohydrates, 18g fat, 3.6g fiber, 21mg cholesterol, 442mg sodium, 356mg potassium.

Pulled Pork Hash with Eggs

Prep time: 10 minutes | **Cook time:** 15 minutes | **Yield:** 4 servings

Ingredients:

- 4 eggs
- 10 oz keto pulled pork, shredded
- 1 teaspoon coconut oil
- 1 teaspoon hot
- pepper
- 1 teaspoon fresh cilantro, chopped
- 1 tomato, chopped
- ¼ cup of water

Method:

1. Melt the coconut oil in the slow cooker on saute mode.
2. Then add keto pulled pork, hot pepper, cilantro, water, and chopped tomato.
3. Cook the ingredients for 5 minutes.
4. Then stir it well with the help of the spatula and crack the eggs over it.
5. Close the lid.
6. Cook the meal on manual mode (high pressure) for 7 minutes. Then make a quick pressure release.

Nutritional info per serve: 267 calories, 22.2g protein, 3.8g carbohydrates, 18.2g fat, 0.3g fiber, 227mg cholesterol, 392mg sodium, 284mg potassium.

Cheese Roll-Ups

Prep time: 10 minutes | **Cook time:** 10 minutes | **Yield:** 3 servings

Ingredients:

- 3 turkey lunch meat slices
- 3 oz Cheddar cheese, grated
- ½ teaspoon minced garlic
- 1 tablespoon cream cheese
- ½ teaspoon coconut oil, melted

Method:

1. Heat the coconut oil on saute mode.
2. Then place the turkey slices in the hot oil and cook them for 5 minutes from each side.
3. Meanwhile, in the mixing bowl mix up cream cheese, minced garlic, and Cheddar cheese.
4. Transfer the cooked turkey slices to the plate and spread them with a cheese mixture.
5. Roll up the turkey slices and secure them with the toothpicks.

Nutritional info per serve: 193 calories, 18.3g protein, 1.6g carbohydrates, 12.3g fat, 0g fiber, 53mg cholesterol, 686mg sodium, 34mg potassium.

Breakfast Taco Skillet

Prep time: 10 minutes | **Cook time:** 17 minutes | **Yield:** 6 servings

Ingredients:

- ½ avocado, chopped
- 3 jalapeno peppers, chopped
- 2 cups ground beef
- 1 teaspoon chili flakes
- 1/3 cup organic almond milk
- ¾ cup black olives, sliced
- 1 teaspoon avocado oil
- 2 eggs, beaten

Method:

1. Melt the avocado oil on saute mode for 2 minutes.
2. Then add ground beef and chili flakes.
3. Cook the meat on saute mode for 4 minutes. Stir it well.
4. Add jalapeno peppers, almond milk, olives, and eggs,
5. Stir the mixture until homogenous.
6. Add chopped avocado and close the lid.
7. Cook the meal on manual mode (high pressure) for 10 minutes. Then make a quick pressure release.

Nutritional info per serve: 148 calories, 6.2g protein, 3.9g carbohydrates, 12.6g fat, 2.2g fiber, 67mg cholesterol, 366mg sodium, 159mg potassium.

Kale and Eggs Bake

Prep time: 10 minutes | **Cook time:** 10 minutes | **Yield:** 2 servings

Ingredients:
- ½ cup kale, chopped
- 3 eggs, beaten
- 1 tablespoon coconut milk
- 1 teaspoon avocado
- oil
- ¼ teaspoon ground black pepper
- 1 cup water, for cooking

Method:
1. In the mixing bowl, mix up chopped kale, eggs, coconut milk, and ground black pepper.
2. Grease the ramekins with avocado oil.
3. Pour the kale-egg mixture in the ramekins and flatten it with the help of the spatula, if needed.
4. Pour water and insert the trivet in the slow cooker.
5. Put the ramekins with egg mixture on the trivet and close the lid.
6. Cook the breakfast on manual mode (high pressure) for 10 minutes. Make a quick pressure release.

Nutritional info per serve: 124 calories, 9g protein, 3g carbohydrates, 8.7g fat, 0.6g fiber, 246mg cholesterol, 101mg sodium, 201mg potassium.

Egg Cups on the Run

Prep time: 10 minutes | **Cook time:** 6 minutes | **Yield:** 3 servings

Ingredients:
- 3 eggs, beaten
- 1 oz tomato, chopped
- 1 oz celery stalk, chopped
- 1 tablespoon scallions, chopped
- 3 oz Cheddar cheese, shredded
- ½ cup coconut milk
- ¼ teaspoon chili flakes
- 1 cup water, for cooking

Method:
1. In the mixing bowl, mix up eggs, tomato, celery stalk, scallions cheese, coconut milk, and chili flakes.
2. Then pour the mixture into the glass cups.
3. Pour water and insert the steamer rack into the slow cooker.
4. Then place the glass cups with egg mixture on the rack. Close and seal the lid.
5. Cook the meal on manual (high pressure) for 6 minutes. Make a quick pressure release.

Nutritional info per serve: 273 calories, 13.7g protein, 3.7g carbohydrates, 23.4g fat, 1.2g fiber, 139mg cholesterol, 252mg sodium, 245mg potassium.

Margherita Egg Cups

Prep time: 10 minutes | **Cook time:** 5 minutes | **Yield:** 2 servings

Ingredients:
- 2 eggs
- 4 oz Mozzarella, shredded
- ½ tomato, chopped
- 1 teaspoon coconut
- oil, melted
- ½ teaspoon dried basil
- 1 cup water, for cooking

Method:
1. Grease the small ramekins with melted coconut oil and crack the eggs inside.
2. Then top the eggs with chopped tomato, basil, and Mozzarella.
3. Pour water and insert the steamer rack into the slow cooker.
4. Place the ramekins with eggs on the rack. Close and seal the lid.
5. Cook the meal on manual (high pressure) for 5 minutes. Allow the natural pressure release for 5 minutes.

Nutritional info per serve: 245 calories, 21.7g protein, 3g carbohydrates, 16.7g fat, 0.2g fiber, 194mg cholesterol, 402mg sodium, 96mg potassium.

Chicken Strips

Prep time: 10 minutes | **Cook time:** 15 minutes | **Yield:** 5 servings

Ingredients:
- 1-pound chicken fillet
- ½ teaspoon ground turmeric
- ½ teaspoon ground black pepper
- 2 tablespoons coconut milk
- 1 cup of organic almond milk
- 1 teaspoon coconut oil, melted

Method:
1. Cut the chicken fillet into the strips and sprinkle with ground turmeric, ground black pepper, and coconut milk.
2. Preheat the coconut oil on saute mode for 3 minutes,
3. Then place the chicken strips in hot oil in one layer. Cook them for 1 minute from each side and add almond milk.
4. Close and seal the lid.
5. Cook the chicken strips on Manual (high pressure) for 10 minutes. Make a quick pressure release.

Nutritional info per serve: 203 calories, 26.6g protein, 1g carbohydrates, 9.7g fat, 0.4g fiber, 81mg cholesterol, 115mg sodium, 282mg potassium.

Coconut Eggs

Prep time: 10 minutes | **Cook time:** 10 minutes | **Yield:** 4 servings

Ingredients:
- 1 teaspoon garlic powder
- 2 tablespoons coconut oil, softened
- 1 teaspoon ground paprika
- 6 eggs, hard-boiled

Method:
1. Peel and cut the eggs into halves.
2. Then melt coconut oil in the slow cooker on Saute mode and add egg halves and roast them for 1 minute.
3. Sprinkle the eggs with garlic powder and ground paprika.

Nutritional info per serve: 157 calories, 8.5g protein, 1.3g carbohydrates, 13.4g fat, 0.3g fiber, 246mg cholesterol, 93mg sodium, 109mg potassium.

Sausage Sandwich

Prep time: 10 minutes | **Cook time:** 30 minutes | **Yield:** 4 servings

Ingredients:
- 4 eggs
- 1 tablespoon coconut oil, softened
- 1 teaspoon white pepper
- 8 lettuce leaves
- 4 sausages, homemade

Method:
1. Toss the coconut oil into the pan and melt it.
2. Crack the eggs inside and add sausages. Sprinkle the sausages with white pepper.
3. Close the lid and cook the ingredients for 30 minutes on High (Manual mode). Make a quick pressure release and open the lid.
4. Then put the eggs and sausages on the lettuce leaves.

Nutritional info per serve: 186 calories, 10.9g protein, 1g carbohydrates, 15.5g fat, 0.2g fiber, 186mg cholesterol, 265mg sodium, 159mg potassium.

Beef Bowl

Prep time: 15 minutes | **Cook time:** 20 minutes | **Yield:** 1 serving

Ingredients:
- 4 ounces ground beef
- 1 oz avocado, chopped
- 1 tomato, chopped
- 1 tablespoon coconut
- oil
- 1 teaspoon white pepper
- 2 oz fresh cilantro, chopped

Method:
1. Put coconut oil in the slow cooker bowl and melt it into Saute mode.
2. Add ground beef and add white pepper and cilantro.
3. Cook the ground beef for 10 minutes on Saute mode. Then stir it well and cook for 5 minutes more on Saute mode.
4. Transfer the meat to the bowls and top with tomato and avocado.

Nutritional info per serve: 415 calories, 36.9g protein, 8.3g carbohydrates, 26.7g fat, 4.8g fiber, 101mg cholesterol, 106mg sodium, 1063mg potassium.

Keto Coffee

Prep time: 5 minutes | **Cook time:** 15 minutes | **Yield:** 2 servings

Ingredients:
- 2 teaspoons instant coffee
- 1 cup of water
- 1/3 cup coconut oil

Method:
1. Pour water into the slow cooker and add coconut oil.
2. Bring the liquid to boil in Saute mode.
3. Then pour the hot liquid into the cups and add instant coffee. Stir the drink well.

Nutritional info per serve: 313 calories, 0g protein, 0g carbohydrates, 36.3g fat, 0g fiber, 0mg cholesterol, 4mg sodium, 4mg potassium.

Seafood Mix

Prep time: 10 minutes | **Cook time:** 5 hours | **Yield:** 3 servings

Ingredients:
- 4 bacon slices, chopped, cooked
- 4 ounces salmon, chopped
- 4 ounces shrimp, peeled
- 1 cup coconut cream

Method:
1. Pour coconut cream into the slow cooker bowl and preheat it on Milk mode/Saute mode until it is hot.
2. Add bacon, salmon, and shrimps.
3. Close the lid and cook the meal on Low for 5 hours.

Nutritional info per serve: 416 calories, 27.2g protein, 5.4g carbohydrates, 32.6g fat, 1.8g fiber, 124cholesterol, 706mg sodium, 563mg potassium.

Vanilla Pancakes

Prep time: 10 minutes | **Cook time:** 10 minutes | **Yield:** 4 servings

Ingredients:

- 1.5 cups almond flour
- 1 teaspoon vanilla extract
- 3 eggs, beaten
- 1 teaspoon baking powder
- 1 teaspoon Erythritol
- 2 tablespoons avocado oil

Method:

1. Pour the coconut oil into the slow cooker bowl and heat it well on Saute mode.
2. Meanwhile, mix all remaining ingredients in the bowl and whisk until smooth.
3. Pour the small amount (2 tablespoons) of the coconut flour mixture in the hot coconut oil and flatten in the shape of the pancake.
4. Roast the pancakes for 1 minute per side on Saute mode.
5. Repeat the same steps with all remaining pancake batter.

Nutritional info per serve: 121 calories, 6.5g protein, 4.9g carbohydrates, 9.4g fat, 1.5g fiber, 123mg cholesterol, 51mg sodium, 194mg potassium.

Easy Eggs Benedict

Prep time: 10 minutes | **Cook time:** 1 minute | **Yield:** 3 servings

Ingredients:

- 3 eggs
- 3 turkey bacon slices, fried
- 1 teaspoon coconut oil
- 1 cup of water

Method:

1. Grease the egg molds with coconut oil and crack eggs inside.
2. Pour water into the slow cooker and insert the rack.
3. Then place the cracked eggs in the rack and close the lid.
4. Cook the eggs for 1 minute on Manual mode (high pressure).
5. Then make a quick pressure release and transfer the eggs to the plate.
6. Top the eggs with bacon slices.

Nutritional info per serve: 96 calories, 8.6g protein, 0.3g carbohydrates, 6.4g fat, 0g fiber, 104mg cholesterol, 184mg sodium, 60mg potassium.

Eggs Bake

Prep time: 10 minutes | **Cook time:** 30 minutes | **Yield:** 4 servings

Ingredients:

- 8 eggs, beaten
- 1 cup Cheddar cheese, shredded
- 1 teaspoon chili flakes
- 1 cup spinach, chopped
- 4 teaspoons avocado oil
- ½ teaspoon onion powder
- 1 cup of water, for cooking

Method:

1. Grease the ramekins with avocado oil
2. Then mix Cheddar cheese with eggs, chili flakes, spinach, and onion powder.
3. Pour the mixture into the ramekins and cover with foil.
4. Pour water into the slow cooker and insert rack.
5. Place the ramekins with eggs on the rack and close the lid.
6. Cook the meal on High for 30 minutes. Then make a natural pressure release and remove the ramekins from the slow cooker.

Nutritional info per serve: 249 calories, 18.4g protein, 1.8g carbohydrates, 18.7g fat, 0.4g fiber, 357mg cholesterol, 305mg sodium, 206mg potassium.

Eggs in Rings

Prep time: 10 minutes | **Cook time:** 10 minutes | **Yield:** 4 servings

Ingredients:

- 1 bell pepper, trimmed
- 4 eggs
- ½ teaspoon olive oil
- ¼ teaspoon chili powder

Method:

1. Slice the bell pepper into 4 rings.
2. Preheat the olive oil in the slow cooker on Saute mode for 1 minute.
3. After this, add bell pepper rings and roast them for 1 minute.
4. Flip the pepper rings on another side.
5. Crack the eggs inside pepper rings and sprinkle with chili powder.
6. Cook the eggs for 5 minutes more on Saute mode.

Nutritional info per serve: 78 calories, 5.9g protein, 2.7g carbohydrates, 5.1g fat, 0.5g fiber, 164mg cholesterol, 64mg sodium, 118mg potassium.

Creamy Omelet Roll

Prep time: 15 minutes | **Cook time:** 20 minutes | **Yield:** 4 servings

Ingredients:

- 8 eggs, whisked
- ¼ cup coconut milk
- 2 oz scallions, chopped
- 1 teaspoon ground paprika
- 1 teaspoon ground black pepper
- 2 oz Cheddar cheese, shredded
- 2 tablespoons avocado oil

Method:

1. Preheat the avocado oil in the slow cooker on Saute mode until it is hot.
2. In the mixing bowl, mix eggs with coconut milk.
3. Separate the mixture into 4 servings.
4. Pour the first part of the mixture in the avocado oil and cook for 2 minutes per side on Saute mode. Repeat the same steps with all remaining egg mixture.
5. Then sprinkle every egg pancake with scallions, ground paprika, ground black pepper, and cheese.
6. Roll the egg pancakes.

Nutritional info per serve: 234 calories, 15.4g protein, 3.8g carbohydrates, 18g fat, 1.4g fiber, 342mg cholesterol, 216mg sodium, 252mg potassium.

Mushroom Scramble

Prep time: 10 minutes | **Cook time:** 15 minutes | **Yield:** 2 servings

Ingredients:

- 1 cup white mushrooms, chopped
- 5 eggs, beaten
- 2 tablespoons avocado oil

Method:

1. Put coconut oil in the slow cooker bowl and melt it into Saute mode.
2. Add mushrooms. Roast the mushrooms for 5-10 minutes on Saute mode. Stir the vegetables from time to time.
3. Then add beaten eggs and carefully stir the mixture.
4. Cook the scramble on High (Manual mode) for 15 minutes. Then make quick pressure release.

Nutritional info per serve: 183 calories, 15.1g protein, 2.8g carbohydrates, 12.8g fat, 1g fiber, 409mg cholesterol, 157mg sodium, 303mg potassium.

Bacon Muffins

Prep time: 10 minutes | **Cook time:** 6 hours | **Yield:** 4 servings

Ingredients:

- 4 bacon slices, cooked, chopped
- 4 eggs, beaten
- 4 tablespoons coconut flour
- 1 teaspoon chili flakes
- 1 tablespoon coconut oil, melted
- 1 cup water, for cooking

Method:

1. Brush the muffin molds with coconut oil
2. After this, in the mixing bowl, mix eggs with coconut flour, chili flakes, and bacon.
3. Pour the batter into the muffin molds (fill ½ part of every mold).
4. Then insert the trivet into the slow cooker. Add water.
5. Place the muffin molds on the trivet and close the lid.
6. Cook the muffins on Low (manual mode) for 6 hours.

Nutritional info per serve: 230 calories, 14.1g protein, 5.1g carbohydrates, 17g fat, 3g fiber, 185mg cholesterol, 516mg sodium, 167mg potassium.

Bacon and Eggs Rolls

Prep time: 10 minutes | **Cook time:** 20 minutes | **Yield:** 4 servings

Ingredients:

- 8 oz bacon, sliced
- 2 eggs, beaten
- 1 teaspoon avocado oil
- ¼ teaspoon ground paprika
- ½ teaspoon dried cilantro

Method:

1. Pour the avocado oil into the slow cooker bowl and add sliced bacon.
2. Roast the bacon on Saute mode for 2 minutes per side.
3. After this, mix eggs ground paprika, and cilantro.
4. Pour the egg mixture over the bacon and close the lid.
5. Cook the meal on High for 15 minutes.
6. Roll the cooked egg mixture into the roll and cut into the serving.

Nutritional info per serve: 340 calories, 23.8g protein, 1.1g carbohydrates, 26.1g fat, 0.1g fiber, 144mg cholesterol, 134mg sodium, 357mg potassium.

Mozzarella Frittata

Prep time: 10 minutes | **Cook time:** 5 hours | **Yield:** 4 servings

Ingredients:

- 8 eggs, beaten
- ½ teaspoon ground nutmeg
- ½ cup Mozzarella, shredded
- 1 tablespoon organic
- almond milk
- ½ teaspoon ground black pepper
- 1 tablespoon avocado oil

Method:

1. Preheat the avocado oil in the slow cooker on Saute mode for 2 minutes.
2. After this, mix eggs with all remaining ingredients.
3. Close the lid and cook the frittata on Low for 5 hours.

Nutritional info per serve: 151 calories, 12.3g protein, 1.5g carbohydrates, 10.8g fat, 0.4g fiber, 329mg cholesterol, 145mg sodium, 143mg potassium.

Eggs and Beef Pie

Prep time: 15 minutes | **Cook time:** 4 hours | **Yield:** 4 servings

Ingredients:

- ½ spring onion, chopped
- 1 cup ground beef
- 3 tablespoons taco seasoning
- ½ cup fresh cilantro,
- chopped
- 8 eggs
- 1 teaspoon coconut oil, melted
- 1 cup of water, for cooking

Method:

1. Brush the slow cooker pie mold with coconut oil.
2. After this, in the mixing bowl mix chopped spring onion, ground beef, taco seasoning, and cilantro.
3. Carefully mix the mixture and add cracked eggs. Mix it until homogenous.
4. Then transfer the mixture to the prepared mold and flatten.
5. Pour water into the slow cooker mold and insert the rivet.
6. Close the lid and cook the pie on high for 4 hours.

Nutritional info per serve: 182 calories, 16.6g protein, 1.9g carbohydrates, 11.9g fat, 0.1g fiber, 345mg cholesterol, 251mg sodium, 134mg potassium.

Salmon Eggs

Prep time: 10 minutes | **Cook time:** 40 minutes | **Yield:** 2 servings

Ingredients:

- 4 eggs, whisked
- 4 oz salmon fillet, chopped
- 1 tablespoon coconut
- oil
- 1 tablespoon chives, chopped

Method:

1. Melt the coconut oil on saute mode.
2. Add salmon and sprinkle with chives.
3. Roast the fish for 2-3 minutes per side on Saute mode.
4. Then add whisked eggs and close the lid.
5. Cook the meal on High pressure (Manual mode) for 30 minutes. Then make a quick pressure release and transfer the meal to the serving plates.

Nutritional info per serve: 260 calories, 22.1g protein, 0.8g carbohydrates, 19.1g fat, 0g fiber, 352mg cholesterol, 148mg sodium, 340mg potassium.

Cauliflower Cakes

Prep time: 15 minutes | **Cook time:** 15 minutes | **Yield:** 3 servings

Ingredients:

- 1 cup cauliflower, shredded
- 5 oz Cheddar cheese, shredded
- 3 eggs, beaten
- 1 teaspoon ground black pepper
- 1 tablespoon coconut flour

Method:

1. In the mixing bowl mix cauliflower with Cheddar cheese, eggs, ground black pepper, and coconut flour.
2. Make the cauliflower cakes.
3. Preheat the slow cooker bowl on saute mode for 3 minutes.
4. Then place 1 cauliflower cake inside.
5. Cook it on saute mode for 3 minutes per side or until it is light brown.
6. Then repeat the same steps with the remaining cauliflower cakes.

Nutritional info per serve: 283 calories, 18.7g protein, 5.8g carbohydrates, 20.8g fat, 2.7g fiber, 213mg cholesterol, 375mg sodium, 215mg potassium.

Avocado Boats

Prep time: 10 minutes | **Cook time:** 30 minutes | **Yield:** 2 servings

Ingredients:
- 1 avocado, cut in half, and pitted
- 2 eggs, beaten
- 1 teaspoon avocado oil
- ½ teaspoon chili flakes
- 1 cup of water, for cooking

Method:
1. Sprinkle the avocado holes with avocado oil and chili flakes.
2. Then pour inside beaten eggs.
3. Pour the water into the slow cooker bowl and insert the trivet.
4. Place the avocado halves on the trivet and close the lid.
5. Cook the avocado boat on High for 30 minutes.

Nutritional info per serve: 268 calories, 7.5g protein, 9g carbohydrates, 24g fat, 6.7g fiber, 164mg cholesterol, 68mg sodium, 547mg potassium.

Cinnamon Eggs

Prep time: 10 minutes | **Cook time:** 10 minutes | **Yield:** 2 servings

Ingredients:
- 4 eggs, hard-boiled, peeled
- 1 teaspoon ground cinnamon
- 1 tablespoon avocado oil
- 1 teaspoon coconut milk

Method:
1. Pour the avocado oil into the slow cooker and preheat it for 2 minutes on Saute mode.
2. Then cut the eggs into halves and put in the hot oil.
3. Sprinkle them with ground cinnamon and coconut milk and cook for 2-3 minutes on Saute mode.

Nutritional info per serve: 144 calories, 11.3g protein, 2.1g carbohydrates, 10.3g fat, 1g fiber, 327mg cholesterol, 124mg sodium, 152mg potassium.

Warm Coconut Smoothie

Prep time: 5 minutes | **Cook time:** 10 minutes | **Yield:** 2 servings

Ingredients:
- 1 cup of coconut milk
- 1 cup fresh spinach, chopped
- 1 cup fresh cilantro, chopped

Method:
1. Put all ingredients in the food processor and blend until smooth.
2. Pour the smoothie into the slow cooker and cook it for 10 minutes on High.
3. Pour the warm smoothie into the serving glasses.

Nutritional info per serve: 281 calories, 3.4g protein, 7.5g carbohydrates, 28.7g fat, 3.2g fiber, 0mg cholesterol, 34mg sodium, 441mg potassium.

Dill Eggs

Prep time: 10 minutes | **Cook time:** 30 minutes | **Yield:** 2 servings

Ingredients:
- 2 eggs
- 1 teaspoon coconut oil
- 1 tablespoon fresh
- dill, chopped
- ¼ teaspoon jalapeno pepper, diced

Method:
1. Put the coconut oil in the slow cooker and melt it on saute mode.
2. Then crack eggs in the coconut oil and sprinkle them with dill and jalapeno.
3. Close the lid and cook the eggs on High for 30 minutes.

Nutritional info per serve: 86 calories, 5.9g protein, 1.2g carbohydrates, 6.7g fat, 0.2g fiber, 164mg cholesterol, 65mg sodium, 111mg potassium.

Chorizo Eggs

Prep time: 10 minutes | **Cook time:** 25 minutes | **Yield:** 4 servings

Ingredients:
- 4 eggs
- 6 oz chorizo, roughly chopped
- 1 tablespoon coconut
- oil
- 1 tomato, chopped
- 1 teaspoon chili powder

Method:
1. Put the chorizo in the slow cooker bowl.
2. Add coconut oil and cook the chorizo on Saute mode for 5 minutes per side.
3. Then stir the chorizo and crack eggs.
4. Add tomato and chili powder.
5. Cook the meal on High for 15 minutes.

Nutritional info per serve: 291 calories, 16g protein, 2.1g carbohydrates, 24.2g fat, 0.4g fiber, 201mg cholesterol, 594mg sodium, 297mg potassium.

Herbed Eggs

Prep time: 10 minutes | **Cook time:** 30 minutes | **Yield:** 4 servings

Ingredients:
- 4 eggs, beaten
- ¼ cup organic almond milk
- 1 cup spinach, chopped
- 1 tablespoon coconut
- oil
- 3 oz Mozzarella, shredded
- 1 teaspoon dried oregano

Method:
1. In the mixing bowl mix eggs with almond milk, spinach, and dried oregano.
2. Melt the coconut oil in the slow cooker bowl on Saute mode and add egg mixture.
3. After this, add mozzarella and close the lid.
4. Cook the meal on High for 30 minutes.

Nutritional info per serve: 190 calories, 12.1g protein, 2.4g carbohydrates, 15.2g fat, 0.7g fiber, 175mg cholesterol, 197mg sodium, 147mg potassium.

Feta Stuffed Chicken

Prep time: 15 minutes | **Cook time:** 17 minutes | **Yield:** 5 servings

Ingredients:
- 1-pound chicken breast, skinless, boneless
- 1 tablespoon Italian seasonings
- 1 teaspoon avocado
- oil
- 3 oz plain Feta cheese, crumbled
- 1 cup water, for cooking

Method:
1. Beat the chicken breast gently with the help of the kitchen hammer.
2. Then make a cut in the breast (to get the pocket).
3. Rub the chicken with Italian seasonings and avocado oil.
4. Then fill the "chicken pocket" with crumbled plain Feta.
5. After this, wrap the chicken breast in the foil.
6. Pour water and insert the steamer rack into the slow cooker.
7. Place the chicken on the rack; close and seal the lid
8. Cook the meal on manual mode (high pressure) for 17 minutes; allow the natural pressure release for 5 minutes.

Nutritional info per serve: 150 calories, 22.3g protein, 1g carbohydrates, 5.7g fat, 0g fiber, 66mg cholesterol, 308mg sodium, 340mg potassium.

Bok Choy Pan

Prep time: 10 minutes | **Cook time:** 30 minutes | **Yield:** 2 servings

Ingredients:
- 6 oz bok choy, sliced
- 1 tablespoon coconut oil, melted
- 2 eggs, beaten
- 1 teaspoon chili powder

Method:
1. Pour the coconut oil into the slow cooker mold.
2. Add sliced bok choy and sprinkle it with chili powder.
3. Roast the bok choy for 4-5 minutes on Saute mode. Stir it occasionally.
4. Then egg eggs and close the lid.
5. Cook the meal on High for 25 minutes.

Nutritional info per serve: 137 calories, 7g protein, 2.9g carbohydrates, 11.6g fat, 1.3g fiber, 164mg cholesterol, 130mg sodium, 298mg potassium.

Cupcake Mugs

Prep time: 20 minutes | **Cook time:** 17 minutes | **Yield:** 6 servings

Ingredients:
- 4 eggs, beaten
- ½ teaspoon ground cinnamon
- ½ teaspoon vanilla extract
- 1 cup coconut flour
- 1 teaspoon baking powder
- 1/3 cup organic almond milk
- 2 tablespoon Erythritol
- 1 teaspoon coconut oil, melted
- 1 cup water, for cooking

Method:
1. Mix up together all ingredients and pour the mixture into the glass jars.
2. Then pour water and insert the steamer rack in the slow cooker.
3. Cover every glass jar with foil and secure the edges.
4. Then place the jars on the rack. Close and seal the lid.
5. Cook the cupcake mugs on Manual (high pressure) for 17 minutes.
6. Then make a quick pressure release and let the cooked meal cool for 10 minutes before serving.

Nutritional info per serve: 175 calories, 8g protein, 14.6g carbohydrates, 10.2g fat, 8.4g fiber,109mg cholesterol, 84mg sodium, 60mg potassium.

Cheesy Fritatta

Prep time: 10 minutes | **Cook time:** 40 minutes | **Yield:** 4 servings

Ingredients:

- 5 eggs, beaten
- 1 tablespoon cream cheese
- 4 jalapeno pepper, sliced
- 3 oz Cheddar cheese, shredded
- ¼ cup coconut milk
- 1 teaspoon avocado oil

Method:

1. Heat the avocado oil in the slow cooker bowl on Saute mode.
2. Then mix eggs with cream cheese and coconut milk.
3. Pour the liquid into the slow cooker and top with jalapeno peppers and cheddar cheese.
4. Close the lid and cook the frittata on High for 35 minutes.

Nutritional info per serve: 213 calories, 12.9g protein, 2.5g carbohydrates, 17.2g fat, 0.8g fiber, 230mg cholesterol, 219mg sodium, 171mg potassium.

Egg Casserole

Prep time: 10 minutes | **Cook time:** 6 hours | **Yield:** 4 servings

Ingredients:

- 8 eggs, beaten
- 1-pound pork sausage, chopped, homemade
- 1 oz Parmesan, grated
- 1 tablespoon avocado oil
- 1 cup water, for cooking

Method:

1. Brush the casserole mold with avocado oil.
2. After this, in the mixing bowl mix eggs with pork sausages.
3. Then pour the mixture into the prepared casserole mold.
4. Top it with Parmesan.
5. Pour water into the slow cooker mold and insert trivet.
6. Place the casserole on the trivet and close the lid.
7. Cook the casserole on Low for 6 hours.

Nutritional info per serve: 538 calories, 35.4g protein, 1.1g carbohydrates, 42.9g fat, 0.2g fiber, 428mg cholesterol, 139mg sodium, 462mg potassium.

Pork Pan

Prep time: 10 minutes | **Cook time:** 20 minutes | **Yield:** 4 servings

Ingredients:

- 1 teaspoon white pepper
- 1 pound minced pork
- 1 tablespoon avocado oil
- ½ teaspoon garlic powder
- 2 oz scallions, chopped

Method:

1. Heat the avocado oil in the slow cooker bowl on Saute mode.
2. Then add minced pork, white pepper, and garlic powder.
3. Cook the mixture for 10-15 minutes on Saute mode.
4. Transfer the cooked pork to the serving pans and top with scallions.

Nutritional info per serve: 174 calories, 30.1g protein, 1.8g carbohydrates, 4.5g fat, 0.7g fiber, 83mg cholesterol, 67mg sodium, 538mg potassium.

Coconut Pancakes

Prep time: 10 minutes | **Cook time:** 15 minutes | **Yield:** 4 servings

Ingredients:

- ½ cup almond flour
- ½ cup coconut flour
- 1 tablespoon coconut shred
- 1 tablespoon Erythritol
- 1 teaspoon baking powder
- ½ teaspoon vanilla extract
- 1 tablespoon avocado oil
- ½ cup coconut milk

Method:

1. Pour avocado oil in the slow cooker bowl and preheat it until hot on Saute mode.
2. Then mix all remaining ingredients in the mixing bowl, stir it until you get a smooth batter.
3. Pour the small amount of batter (2 tablespoons) in the hot avocado oil and flatten it in the shape of a pancake.
4. Roast the pancake on Saute mode for 1 minute per side.
5. Repeat the same steps with all remaining batter.

Nutritional info per serve: 179 calories, 4.5g protein, 10.5g carbohydrates, 13.1g fat, 7.5g fiber, 0mg cholesterol, 38mg sodium, 217mg potassium.

Nut Yogurt

Prep time: 10 minutes | **Cook time:** 6 minutes | **Yield:** 4 servings

Ingredients:

- 1 cup of coconut yogurt
- ½ oz pistachio nuts, chopped
- ½ oz hazelnuts, chopped
- ½ oz macadamia nuts, chopped
- 1 teaspoon Erythritol
- ½ teaspoon coconut oil

Method:

1. Preheat the coconut oil on saute mode for 1 minute.

2. When the oil is hot, add pistachio nuts, hazelnuts, and macadamia nuts. Cook them on saute mode for 5 minutes. Stir the nuts constantly.

3. Then cool the nuts well and mix them up with Erythritol and coconut yogurt.

4. Put the cooked meal in the serving jars and cool well before serving.

Nutritional info per serve: 146 calories, 5g protein, 10.5g carbohydrates, 10.6g fat, 1.2g fiber, 10mg cholesterol, 47mg sodium, 74mg potassium.

Pancetta Eggs

Prep time: 10 minutes | **Cook time:** 5 minutes | **Yield:** 4 servings

Ingredients:

- 2 oz Pancetta, fried
- 4 eggs
- 1 teaspoon scallions, chopped
- Cooking spray
- 1 cup water, for cooking

Method:

1. Spray the egg molds with cooking spray.

2. Crack the eggs in the egg molds and sprinkle with scallions and Pancetta. Stir every egg mixture gently.

3. Then pour water and insert the steamer rack in the slow cooker.

4. Put the egg molds in the slow cooker. Close and seal the lid.

5. Cook the meal on manual mode (high pressure) for 5 minutes. Make a quick pressure release.

Nutritional info per serve: 140 calories, 10.8g protein, 0.6g carbohydrates, 10.3g fat, 0g fiber, 179mg cholesterol, 389mg sodium, 140mg potassium.

Basil Scramble

Prep time: 10 minutes | **Cook time:** 25 minutes | **Yield:** 4 servings

Ingredients:

- 1 teaspoon fresh basil, chopped
- 8 eggs, beaten
- 2 oz bacon, chopped
- 1 teaspoon olive oil

Method:

1. Heat the olive oil in the slow cooker bowl on the Saute mode until hot.

2. Add bacon and roast it for 4-5 minutes per side on Saute mode.

3. Add eggs and fresh basil.

4. Stir the eggs from time to time for 10 minutes or until they are set.

Nutritional info per serve: 213 calories, 16.3g protein, 0.9g carbohydrates, 15.8g fat, 0g fiber, 343mg cholesterol, 451mg sodium, 199mg potassium.

Chili Roasted Eggs

Prep time: 5 minutes | **Cook time:** 7 minutes | **Yield:** 3 servings

Ingredients:

- 1 teaspoon butter
- 3 eggs
- ½ teaspoon chili flakes

Method:

1. Heat butter in the slow cooker on Saute mode.

2. When the butter is hot, crack the eggs in the slow cooker bowl and sprinkle with chili flakes.

3. Cook the eggs in saute mode for 5 minutes.

Nutritional info per serve: 74 calories, 5.6g protein, 0.4g carbohydrates, 5.6g fat, 0g fiber, 167mg cholesterol, 71mg sodium, 60mg potassium.

Meat

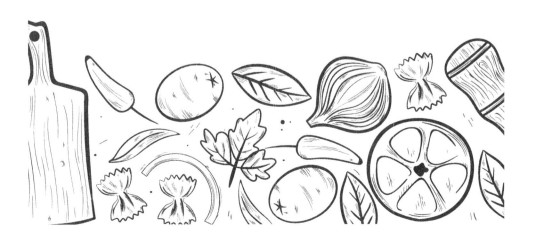

Beef in Sauce

Yield: 4 servings | **Prep time:** 10 minutes | **Cook time:** 9 hours

Ingredients:

- 1-pound beef stew meat, chopped
- 1 teaspoon garam masala
- 1 cup of water
- 1 tablespoon coconut flour
- 1 teaspoon garlic powder
- 1 yellow onion, diced

Method:

1. Whisk coconut flour with water until smooth and pour the liquid into the slow cooker.
2. Add garam masala and beef stew meat.
3. After this, add onion and garlic powder.
4. Close the lid and cook the meat on low for 9 hours.
5. Serve the cooked beef with thick gravy from the slow cooker.

Nutritional info per serve: 231 calories, 35g protein, 4.6g carbohydrates, 7.1g fat, 0.7g fiber, 101mg cholesterol, 79mg sodium, 507mg potassium

Pork Casserole

Yield: 7 servings | **Prep time:** 10 minutes | **Cook time:** 8 hours

Ingredients:

- 1 cup cauliflower, chopped
- 1 teaspoon ground black pepper
- 1 teaspoon cayenne pepper
- 7 oz pork mince
- 1 cup Cheddar cheese, shredded
- ½ cup coconut milk
- 1 teaspoon avocado oil

Method:

1. Brush the slow cooker bowl with avocado oil from inside.
2. Then mix minced pork with ground black pepper and cayenne pepper.
3. Place the meat in the slow cooker and flatten gently.
4. After this, top it with cauliflower and Cheddar cheese.
5. Add coconut milk and close the lid.
6. Cook the casserole on Low for 8 hours.

Nutritional info per serve: 188 calories, 4.8g protein, 14.9g carbohydrates, 10.7g fat, 1.2g fiber, 17mg cholesterol, 107mg sodium, 115mg potassium

Swedish Style Meatballs

Yield: 4 servings | **Prep time:** 10 minutes | **Cook time:** 5.5 hours

Ingredients:

- ½ cup of water
- ½ cup coconut cream
- 1 tablespoon almond flour
- 9 oz minced pork
- 1 teaspoon ground
- black pepper
- 1 tablespoon coconut shred
- 1 tablespoon fresh parsley, chopped

Method:

1. Make the meatballs: mix minced pork with ground black pepper and coconut shred.
2. Make the small meatballs and place them in the slow cooker in one layer.
3. After this, mix water with coconut cream and almond flour.
4. Pour the liquid over the meatballs and cook them on High for 5.5 hours.

Nutritional info per serve: 126 calories, 17.5g protein, 4.1g carbohydrates, 4.1g fat, 0.3g fiber, 52mg cholesterol, 642mg sodium, 297mg potassium.

Cilantro Meatballs

Yield: 6 servings | **Prep time:** 20 minutes | **Cook time:** 4 hours

Ingredients:

- 1-pound minced beef
- 1 teaspoon minced garlic
- 1 egg, beaten
- 1 teaspoon chili flakes
- 2 teaspoons dried cilantro
- 1 tablespoon almond flour
- ½ cup of water
- 1 tablespoon avocado oil

Method:

1. In the bowl mix minced beef, garlic, egg, chili flakes, cilantro, and almond flour.
2. Then make the meatballs.
3. After this, heat the avocado oil in the skillet.
4. Cook the meatballs in the hot oil on high heat for 1 minute per side.
5. Transfer the roasted meatballs to the slow cooker, add water, and close the lid.
6. Cook the meatballs on High for 4 hours.

Nutritional info per serving: 178 calories, 24.1g protein, 1.5g carbohydrates, 7.7g fat, 0.1g fiber, 95mg cholesterol, 61mg sodium, 321mg potassium.

Beef and Chives Bowl

Yield: 4 servings | **Prep time:** 10 minutes | **Cook time:** 5 hours

Ingredients:

- 1 teaspoon chili powder
- 2 oz chives, chopped
- 1-pound beef stew meat, cubed
- 1 cup of water
- 2 tablespoons keto tomato paste
- 1 teaspoon minced garlic

Method:

1. Mix water with tomato paste and pour the liquid into the slow cooker.
2. Add chili powder, beef, and minced garlic.
3. Close the lid and cook the meal on high for 5 hours.
4. When the meal is cooked, transfer the mixture to the bowls and top with chives.

Nutritional info per serve: 258 calories, 36.4g protein, 10.4g carbohydrates, 7.7g fat, 2g fiber, 101mg cholesterol, 99mg sodium, 697mg potassium.

Cheese and Pork Casserole

Yield: 5 servings | **Prep time:** 40 minutes | **Cook time:** 6 hours

Ingredients:

- 2 cups ground pork
- 1 cup Cheddar cheese, shredded
- ½ cup organic almond milk
- 1 teaspoon dried cilantro
- ½ teaspoon chili powder
- 1 tablespoon coconut oil, softened
- 1 cup of water, for cooking

Method:

1. Grease the casserole mold with coconut oil
2. After this, mix ground pork with dried cilantro, almond milk, and chili powder.
3. Put the mixture in the casserole mold, flatten it in one layer, and top with Cheddar cheese.
4. Pour water into the slow cooker and insert the rack inside.
5. Place the casserole mold on the rack and close the lid.
6. Cook the meal on Low for 6 hours.

Nutritional info per serve: 356 calories, 22.3g protein, 1.8g carbohydrates, 29g fat, 0.6g fiber, 83mg cholesterol, 192mg sodium, 317mg potassium.

Ground Pork Pie

Yield: 6 servings | **Prep time:** 25 minutes | **Cook time:** 7 hours

Ingredients:

- 1 cup coconut flour
- 3 tablespoons Psyllium husk
- 2 tablespoons coconut oil, softened
- 1 cup ground pork
- 2 oz scallions, chopped
- 1 tablespoon almond flour
- 1 teaspoon chili powder
- 1 teaspoon avocado oil
- 1 cup of water, for cooking

Method:

1. In the mixing bowl, mix coconut flour, psyllium husk, coconut oil, and almond flour. Knead the dough.
2. After this, put the dough in the baking pan and flatten it in the shape of the pie crust with the help of the finger palms.
3. After this, in the mixing bowl, mix ground pork with scallions, chili powder, and avocado oil.
4. Put the mixture over the pie crust and flatten well.
5. Pour water into the slow cooker and insert trivet inside.
6. Place the pie on the trivet and close the lid.
7. Cook the pie on Low for 7 hours.

Nutritional info per serve: 362 calories, 18.6g protein, 30.9g carbohydrates, 21.2g fat, 23g fiber, 49mg cholesterol, 128mg sodium, 229mg potassium.

Onion Beef

Yield: 14 servings | **Prep time:** 10 minutes | **Cook time:** 5.5 hours

Ingredients:

- 4-pounds beef sirloin, sliced
- 2 cups yellow onion, chopped
- 3 cups of water
- ½ cup coconut oil
- 1 teaspoon ground black pepper
- 1 bay leaf

Method:

1. Mix beef sirloin with ground black pepper and transfer in the slow cooker.
2. Add coconut oil, water, onion, and bay leaf.
3. Close the lid and cook the meat on High for 5.5 hours.

Nutritional info per serve: 306 calories, 39.6g protein, 1.7g carbohydrates, 14.7g fat, 0.4g fiber, 133mg cholesterol, 301mg sodium, 551mg potassium.

Balsamic Beef

Yield: 4 servings | **Prep time:** 15 minutes | **Cook time:** 9 hours

Ingredients:
- 1-pound beef stew meat, cubed
- 1 teaspoon cayenne pepper
- 4 tablespoons apple
- cider vinegar
- ½ cup of water
- 2 tablespoons coconut oil

Method:
1. Toss the coconut oil in the slow cooker and melt it on Saute mode.
2. Then add meat and roast it for 2 minutes per side on Saute mode.
3. Add apple cider vinegar, cayenne pepper, and water.
4. Close the lid and cook the meal on Low for 9 hours.

Nutritional info per serve: 266 calories, 34.5g protein, 0.4g carbohydrates, 12.9g fat, 0.1g fiber, 117mg cholesterol, 117mg sodium, 479mg potassium.

Hawaiian Meatballs in Raspberry Sauce

Yield: 4 servings | **Prep time:** 15 minutes | **Cook time:** 5 hours

Ingredients:
- 12 oz ground pork
- 1 oz raspberries, mashed
- 1 teaspoon dried cilantro
- 1 teaspoon chili
- flakes
- 1 tablespoon coconut flour
- 1 cup water
- 2 tablespoons coconut oil

Method:
1. In the mixing bowl mix ground pork, dried cilantro, and chili flakes.
2. Make the small meatballs.
3. Then put the coconut oil in the skillet and melt it.
4. Add the meatballs and roast them for 2 minutes per side.
5. Transfer the roasted meatballs to the slow cooker.
6. Mix mashed raspberries with coconut flour and water, and pour the liquid into the slow cooker.
7. Cook the meatballs on low for 5 hours.

Nutritional info per serve: 196 calories, 22.6g protein, 5.5g carbohydrates, 8.8g fat, 0.1g fiber, 77mg cholesterol, 381mg sodium, 404mg potassium

Turmeric Beef Brisket

Yield: 5 servings | **Prep time:** 10 minutes | **Cook time:** 5 hours

Ingredients:
- 12 oz beef brisket, chopped
- 1 tablespoon ground turmeric
- 1 teaspoon chili powder
- ½ teaspoon garlic powder
- 1 cup of water
- 1 tablespoon coconut oil

Method:
1. Toss the coconut oil in the skillet and melt it.
2. Meanwhile, mix the meat with ground turmeric, chili powder, and garlic powder.
3. Put the meat in the hot oil and roast it for 2 minutes per side on high heat.
4. After this, pour water into the slow cooker.
5. Add roasted meat and close the lid.
6. Cook the meal on High for 5 hours.

Nutritional info per serve: 157 calories, 20.9g protein, 1.4g carbohydrates, 7.2g fat, 0.5g fiber, 61mg cholesterol, 52mg sodium, 322mg potassium.

Leek Stuffed Beef

Yield: 2 servings | **Prep time:** 20 minutes | **Cook time:** 7 hours

Ingredients:
- 8 oz beef tenderloin
- 4 oz leek, chopped
- 1 teaspoon coconut oil
- 1 tablespoon dried parsley
- 1 oz bacon, chopped
- 1 teaspoon avocado oil

Method:
1. Cut the beef tenderloin into 2 servings.
2. Then mix leek with dried parsley, and chopped bacon.
3. Spread the mixture over the beef tenderloins. Fold the meat and secure it with the help of the toothpicks.
4. Mix coconut oil with avocado oil and put it in the slow cooker.
5. Preheat the mixture until hot on Saute mode.
6. After this, add beef rolls and close the lid.
7. Cook the meal on Low for 7 hours.

Nutritional info per serve: 368 calories, 39g protein, 8.5g carbohydrates, 19g fat, 1.2g fiber, 120mg cholesterol, 407mg sodium, 605mg potassium.

Mustard Beef

Yield: 4 servings | **Prep time:** 10 minutes | **Cook time:** 8 hours

Ingredients:
- 1-pound beef sirloin, chopped
- 1 tablespoon capers, drained
- 1 cup of water
- 2 tablespoons mustard
- 1 tablespoon coconut oil

Method:
1. Mix meat with mustard and leave for 10 minutes to marinate.
2. Then melt the coconut oil in the skillet.
3. Add meat and roast it for 1 minute per side on high heat.
4. After this, transfer the meat to the slow cooker.
5. Add water and capers.
6. Cook the meal on Low for 8 hours.

Nutritional info per serve: 267 calories, 35.9g protein, 2.1g carbohydrates, 12.1g fat, 0.9g fiber, 101mg cholesterol, 140mg sodium, 496mg potassium.

Sweet Beef

Yield: 4 servings | **Prep time:** 10 minutes | **Cook time:** 5 hours

Ingredients:
- 1-pound beef roast, sliced
- 1 tablespoon Erythritol
- 2 tablespoons lemon juice
- 1 teaspoon dried oregano
- 1 cup of water

Method:
1. Mix water with Erythritol, lemon juice, and dried oregano.
2. Then pour the liquid into the slow cooker.
3. Add beef roast and close the lid.
4. Cook the meal on High for 5 hours.

Nutritional info per serve: 227 calories, 34.5g protein, 3.8g carbohydrates, 7.2g fat, 0.2g fiber, 101mg cholesterol, 78mg sodium, 483mg potassium.

Beef and Sauerkraut Bowl

Yield: 4 servings | **Prep time:** 10 minutes | **Cook time:** 5 hours

Ingredients:
- 1 cup sauerkraut
- 1-pound corned beef, chopped
- ¼ cup apple cider vinegar
- 1 cup of water

Method:
1. Pour water and apple cider vinegar into the slow cooker.
2. Add corned beef and cook it on High for 5 hours.
3. Then chop the meat roughly and put it in the serving bowls.
4. Top the meat with sauerkraut.

Nutritional info per serving: 202 calories, 15.5g protein, 1.7g carbohydrates, 14.2g fat, 1g fiber, 71mg cholesterol, 1240mg sodium, 236mg potassium.

Beef with Greens

Yield: 3 servings | **Prep time:** 15 minutes | **Cook time:** 8 hours

Ingredients:
- 1 cup fresh spinach, chopped
- 9 oz beef stew meat, cubed
- 1 cup swiss chard, chopped
- 2 cups of water
- 1 teaspoon coconut oil
- 1 teaspoon dried rosemary

Method:
1. Put the coconut oil in the slow cooker bowl and preheat it until it is melted on Saute mode.
2. Add beef and roast it for 1 minute per side on Saute mode.
3. Add swiss chard, spinach, water, and rosemary.
4. Close the lid and cook the meal on Low for 8 hours.

Nutritional info per serve: 177 calories, 26.3g protein, 1.1g carbohydrates, 7g fat, 0.6g fiber, 76mg cholesterol, 95mg sodium, 449mg potassium.

Stuffed Jalapenos

Yield: 3 servings | **Prep time:** 10 minutes | **Cook time:** 4.5 hours

Ingredients:
- 6 jalapenos, deseed
- 4 oz minced beef
- 1 teaspoon garlic powder
- ½ cup of water

Method:
1. Mix the minced beef with garlic powder.
2. Then fill the jalapenos with minced meat and arrange it in the slow cooker.
3. Add water and cook the jalapenos on High for 4.5 hours.

Nutritional info per serve: 55 calories, 7.5g protein, 2.3g carbohydrates, 1.9g fat, 0.9g fiber, 0mg cholesterol, 2mg sodium, 71mg potassium.

Cilantro Beef

Yield: 4 servings | **Prep time:** 10 minutes | **Cook time:** 4.5 hours

Ingredients:
- 1-pound beef loin, roughly chopped
- ¼ cup apple cider vinegar
- 1 tablespoon dried cilantro
- ½ teaspoon dried basil
- 1 cup of water
- 1 teaspoon keto tomato paste

Method:
1. Mix meat with keto tomato paste, dried cilantro, and basil.
2. Then transfer it to the slow cooker.
3. Add apple cider vinegar and water.
4. Cook the cilantro beef for 4.5 hours on High.

Nutritional info per serve: 211 calories, 30.4g protein, 0.4g carbohydrates, 9.5g fat, 0.1g fiber, 81mg cholesterol, 66mg sodium, 412mg potassium.

Beef and Artichokes Bowls

Yield: 4 servings | **Prep time:** 10 minutes | **Cook time:** 7 hours

Ingredients:
- 6 oz beef sirloin, chopped
- ½ teaspoon cayenne pepper
- ½ teaspoon white pepper
- 4 artichoke hearts, chopped
- 1 cup of water

Method:
1. Mix meat with white pepper and cayenne pepper. Transfer it to the slow cooker bowl.
2. Add artichoke hearts and water.
3. Close the lid and cook the meal on Low for 7 hours.

Nutritional info per serve: 157 calories, 18.3g protein, 17.3g carbohydrates, 2.9g fat, 8.9g fiber, 38mg cholesterol, 182mg sodium, 789mg potassium.

Beef Masala

Yield: 6 servings | **Prep time:** 15 minutes | **Cook time:** 9 hours

Ingredients:
- 1-pound beef sirloin, sliced
- 1 teaspoon garam masala
- 2 tablespoons lemon juice
- 1 teaspoon ground paprika
- ½ cup of organic almond milk
- 1 teaspoon dried mint

Method:
1. In the bowl mix almond milk with dried mint, ground paprika, lemon juice, and garam masala.
2. Then add beef sirloin and mix the mixture. Leave it for at least 10 minutes to marinate.
3. Then transfer the mixture to the slow cooker.
4. Cook it on Low for 9 hours.

Nutritional info per serve: 283 calories, 35.3g protein, 2.2g carbohydrates, 14.4g fat, 0.9g fiber, 101mg cholesterol, 82mg sodium, 560mg potassium.

Beef Saute with Endives

Yield: 4 servings | **Prep time:** 10 minutes | **Cook time:** 8 hours

Ingredients:
- 1-pound beef sirloin, chopped
- 3 oz endives, roughly chopped
- 1 teaspoon peppercorns
- 1 onion, sliced
- 1 cup of water

Method:
1. Mix beef with onion and peppercorns.
2. Place the mixture in the slow cooker.
3. Add water.
4. Then close the lid and cook it on High for 5 hours.
5. After this, add endives and cook the meal for 3 hours on Low.

Nutritional info per serve: 238 calories, 35.4g protein, 6.4g carbohydrates, 7.2g fat, 1.9g fiber, 101mg cholesterol, 175mg sodium, 689mg potassium.

Keto Turkish Meat Saute

Yield: 4 servings | **Prep time:** 10 minutes | **Cook time:** 10 hours

Ingredients:
- 1 cup green peas
- 1 cup cauliflower, chopped
- 2 cups of water
- 10 oz beef sirloin,
- chopped
- 1 teaspoon ground black pepper
- 1 tablespoon keto tomato paste

Method:
1. Put all ingredients in the slow cooker and carefully mix.
2. Then close the lid.
3. Cook the saute on Low for 10 hours.

Nutritional info per serve: 192 calories, 24.3g protein, 12.2g carbohydrates, 4.7g fat, 3.1g fiber, 63mg cholesterol, 640mg sodium, 575mg potassium.

Thyme Beef

Yield: 2 servings | **Prep time:** 15 minutes | **Cook time:** 5 hours

Ingredients:

- 8 oz beef sirloin, chopped
- 1 tablespoon dried thyme
- 1 tablespoon coconut oil, melted
- ½ cup of water

Method:

1. Preheat the skillet well.
2. Then mix beef with dried thyme and coconut oil.
3. Put the meat in the hot skillet and roast for 2 minutes per side on high heat.
4. Then transfer the meat to the slow cooker.
5. Add water.
6. Cook the meal on High for 5 hours.

Nutritional info per serve: 274 calories, 34.5g protein, 0.9g carbohydrates, 14.2g fat, 0.5g fiber, 101mg cholesterol, 1240mg sodium, 469mg potassium.

Hot Beef

Yield: 4 servings | **Prep time:** 15 minutes | **Cook time:** 8 hours

Ingredients:

- 1-pound beef sirloin, chopped
- 2 tablespoons keto hot sauce
- 1 tablespoon coconut oil, melted
- ½ cup of water

Method:

1. In the shallow bowl mix keto hot sauce with coconut oil.
2. Then mix beef sirloin with hot sauce mixture and leave for 10 minutes to marinate.
3. Put the marinated beef in the slow cooker.
4. Add water and close the lid.
5. Cook the meal on Low for 8 hours.

Nutritional info per serve: 241 calories, 34.4g protein, 0.1g carbohydrates, 10.6g fat, 0g fiber, 101mg cholesterol, 266mg sodium, 467mg potassium.

Spiced Beef

Yield: 4 servings | **Prep time:** 10 minutes | **Cook time:** 9 hours

Ingredients:

- 1-pound beef loin
- 1 teaspoon allspice
- 1 teaspoon olive oil
- 1 tablespoon minced onion
- 1 cup of water

Method:

1. Rub the beef loin with allspice, olive oil, and minced onion.
2. Put the meat in the slow cooker.
3. Add water and close the lid.
4. Cook the beef on Low for 9 hours.
5. When the meat is cooked, slice it into servings.

Nutritional info per serve: 219 calories, 30.4g protein, 0.6g carbohydrates, 10.7g fat, 0.2g fiber, 81mg cholesterol, 65mg sodium, 395mg potassium.

Beef Chops with Sprouts

Yield: 5 servings | **Prep time:** 10 minutes | **Cook time:** 7 hours

Ingredients:

- 1-pound beef loin
- ½ cup bean sprouts
- 1 cup of water
- 1 tablespoon keto
- tomato paste
- 1 teaspoon chili powder

Method:

1. Cut the beef loin into 5 beef chops and sprinkle the beef chops with chili powder.
2. Then place them in the slow cooker.
3. Add water and keto tomato paste. Cook the meat on low for 7 hours.
4. Then transfer the cooked beef chops to the plates, sprinkle with tomato gravy from the slow cooker, and top with bean sprouts.

Nutritional info per serve: 175 calories,25.2g protein, 1.6g carbohydrates, 7.8g fat, 0.3g fiber, 64mg cholesterol, 526mg sodium, 386mg potassium.

Braised Beef

Yield: 2 servings | **Prep time:** 8 minutes | **Cook time:** 9 hours

Ingredients:

- 8 oz beef tenderloin, chopped
- 1 garlic clove, peeled
- 1 teaspoon
- peppercorn
- 1 tablespoon dried basil
- 2 cups of water

Method:

1. Put all ingredients from the list above in the slow cooker.
2. Gently stir the mixture and close the lid.
3. Cook the beef on low for 9 hours.

Nutritional info per serve: 239 calories, 33.1g protein, 1.2g carbohydrates, 10.4g fat, 0.3g fiber, 104mg cholesterol, 1238mg sodium, 431mg potassium.

Beef Ragout with Eggplant

Yield: 5 servings | **Prep time:** 10 minutes | **Cook time:** 5 hours

Ingredients:
- 1 tablespoon keto tomato paste
- 2 eggplants, peeled, chopped
- 1-pound beef stew meat, chopped
- 1 teaspoon ground black pepper
- 2 cup of water

Method:
1. Pour water into the slow cooker.
2. Add meat and ground black pepper.
3. Cook the mixture on High for 4 hours.
4. Then add tomato paste eggplants. Stir the meal and cook it on high for 1 hour more.

Nutritional info per serve: 227 calories, 29.8g protein, 13.9g carbohydrates, 6.1g fat, 8.1g fiber, 81mg cholesterol, 69mg sodium, 907mg potassium.

Coconut Beef

Yield: 5 servings | **Prep time:** 10 minutes | **Cook time:** 8 hours

Ingredients:
- 1 cup baby spinach, chopped
- 1 cup of organic almond milk
- 1-pound beef tenderloin, chopped
- 1 teaspoon avocado oil
- 1 teaspoon dried rosemary
- 1 teaspoon garlic powder

Method:
1. Roast meat in avocado oil for 1 minute per side on high heat.
2. Ten transfer the meat in the slow cooker.
3. Add garlic powder, dried rosemary, almond milk, and baby spinach.
4. Close the lid and cook the meal on Low for 8 hours.

Nutritional info per serve: 303 calories, 27.6g protein, 3.5g carbohydrates, 19.9g fat, 1.4g fiber, 83mg cholesterol, 66mg sodium, 495mg potassium.

BBQ Beef Short Ribs

Yield: 4 servings | **Prep time:** 10 minutes | **Cook time:** 5 hours

Ingredients:
- 1-pound beef short ribs
- ¼ cup of water
- 1/3 cup keto BBQ sauce
- 1 teaspoon chili powder

Method:
1. Rub the beef short ribs with chili powder and put them in the slow cooker.
2. Mix water with keto BBQ sauce and pour the liquid into the slow cooker.
3. Cook the meat on High for 5 hours.

Nutritional info per serve: 266 calories, 32.8g protein, 7.9g carbohydrates, 10.4g fat, 0.3g fiber, 103mg cholesterol, 308mg sodium, 468mg potassium.

Beef Roast

Yield: 5 servings | **Prep time:** 10 minutes | **Cook time:** 6 hours

Ingredients:
- 1-pound beef chuck roast
- 1 tablespoon keto ketchup
- 1 tablespoon keto mayonnaise
- 1 teaspoon chili powder
- 1 teaspoon olive oil
- 1 teaspoon lemon juice
- ½ cup of water

Method:
1. In the bowl mix ketchup, mayonnaise, chili powder, olive oil, and lemon juice.
2. Then sprinkle the beef chuck roast with a ketchup mixture.
3. Pour the water into the slow cooker.
4. Add beef chuck roast and close the lid.
5. Cook the meat on High for 6 hours.

Nutritional info per serve: 354 calories, 23.9g protein, 1.8g carbohydrates, 27.3g fat, 0.2g fiber, 94mg cholesterol, 119mg sodium, 230mg potassium.

Beef Dip

Yield: 6 servings | **Prep time:** 10 minutes | **Cook time:** 10 hours

Ingredients:
- ½ cup coconut cream
- 1 yellow onion, diced
- 1 teaspoon cream cheese
- ½ cup Cheddar cheese, shredded
- 1 teaspoon garlic powder
- 4 oz dried beef, chopped
- ½ cup of water

Method:
1. Put all ingredients in the slow cooker.
2. Gently stir the ingredients and close the lid.
3. Cook the dip on Low for 10 hours.

Nutritional info per serve: 118 calories, 8.6g protein, 2.5g carbohydrates, 8.2g fat, 0.4g fiber, 41mg cholesterol, 78mg sodium, 126mg potassium.

Lunch Beef

Yield: 2 servings | **Prep time:** 10 minutes | **Cook time:** 8 hours

Ingredients:
- ½ white onion, sliced
- 1 teaspoon Erythritol
- 1 teaspoon chili powder
- 1 teaspoon keto hot
- sauce
- ½ cup okra, chopped
- 1 cup of water
- 7 oz beef loin, chopped

Method:
1. Mix the beef loin with hot sauce, chili powder, and Erythritol.
2. Transfer the meat to the slow cooker.
3. Add water, okra, and onion.
4. Cook the meal on Low for 8 hours.

Nutritional info per serve: 179 calories, 19.3g protein, 7.8g carbohydrates, 7.4g fat, 1.8g fiber, 53mg cholesterol, 520mg sodium, 146mg potassium.

Braised Beef Strips

Yield: 4 servings | **Prep time:** 10 minutes | **Cook time:** 5 hours

Ingredients:
- ½ cup cremini mushroom, sliced
- 1 yellow onion, sliced
- 1 cup of water
- 1 tablespoon coconut
- oil
- 1 teaspoon white pepper
- 10 oz beef loin, cut into strips

Method:
1. Melt the coconut oil in the skillet.
2. Add mushrooms and roast them for 5 minutes on medium heat.
3. Then transfer the mushrooms to the slow cooker.
4. Add all remaining ingredients and close the lid.
5. Cook the meal on High for 5 hours

Nutritional info per serve: 173 calories, 19.6g protein, 3.2g carbohydrates, 9.4g fat, 0.8g fiber, 50mg cholesterol, 624mg sodium, 316mg potassium.

Burgers

Yield: 4 servings | **Prep time:** 10 minutes | **Cook time:** 4 hours

Ingredients:
- 10 oz ground beef
- 1 tablespoon minced onion
- 1 teaspoon dried dill
- 2 tablespoons water
- 1 teaspoon ground black pepper
- 1/3 cup chicken broth

Method:
1. Mix the minced beef with onion, dill, water, and ground black pepper.
2. Make 4 burgers and arrange them in the slow cooker bowl.
3. Add chicken broth and close the lid.
4. Cook the burgers on high for 4 hours.

Nutritional info per serve: 135 calories, 21.7g protein, 0.8g carbohydrates, 4.5g fat, 0.2g fiber, 63mg cholesterol, 111mg sodium, 305mg potassium.

Ginger Beef

Yield: 2 servings | **Prep time:** 10 minutes | **Cook time:** 4.5 hours

Ingredients:
- 10 oz beef brisket, sliced
- 1 teaspoon minced ginger
- 1 teaspoon ground
- coriander
- 1 tablespoon olive oil
- 1 tablespoon lemon juice
- 1 cup of water

Method:
1. In the bowl mix lemon juice and olive oil.
2. Then mix beef brisket with ground coriander and minced ginger.
3. Sprinkle the meat with an oil mixture and transfer to the slow cooker.
4. Add water and cook the meal on High for 4.5 hours.

Nutritional info per serve: 328 calories, 43.1g protein, 0.8g carbohydrates, 15.9g fat, 0.1g fiber, 127mg cholesterol, 99mg sodium, 595mg potassium.

Fall Pork

Yield: 4 servings | **Prep time:** 8 minutes | **Cook time:** 10 hours

Ingredients:
- 9 oz pork tenderloin, chopped
- ½ cup zucchini, chopped
- 2 cups of water
- 2 tomatoes, chopped
- 1 teaspoon Italian seasonings

Method:
1. Put all ingredients in the slow cooker.
2. Close the lid and cook the meal on Low for 10 hours.
3. Carefully mix the cooked meal before serving.

Nutritional info per serve: 119 calories, 17.5g protein, 5.7g carbohydrates, 2.8g fat, 1.8g fiber, 47mg cholesterol, 635mg sodium, 484mg potassium

Aromatic Meatloaf

Yield: 6 servings | **Prep time:** 10 minutes | **Cook time:** 6 hours

Ingredients:
- 1 rutabaga, peeled, grated
- 1 teaspoon garlic powder
- 1 onion, minced
- 10 oz minced beef
- 1 egg, beaten
- 1 teaspoon coconut oil, melted
- 1 cup of water

Method:
1. In the mixing bowl, mix grated rutabaga, garlic powder, minced onion, minced beef, and egg.
2. Then brush the meatloaf mold with coconut oil.
3. Place the minced beef mixture inside and flatten it.
4. Then pour the water into the slow cooker.
5. Place the mold with meatloaf in water.
6. Close the lid and cook the meal on High for 6 hours.

Nutritional info per serve: 130 calories, 16.1g protein, 7.1g carbohydrates, 3.8g fat, 1.1g fiber, 69mg cholesterol, 45mg sodium, 354mg potassium.

Meat and Mushrooms Saute

Yield: 4 servings | **Prep time:** 10 minutes | **Cook time:** 5 hours

Ingredients:
- 8 oz pork sirloin, sliced
- 1 cup white mushrooms, chopped
- 1 onion, sliced
- 1 cup coconut cream
- 1 teaspoon ground black pepper

Method:
1. Put all ingredients in the slow cooker and carefully mix with the help of the spatula.
2. Then close the lid and cook the sauté on High for 5 hours.

Nutritional info per serve: 156 calories, 13g protein, 5.4g carbohydrates, 9g fat, 0.9g fiber, 47mg cholesterol, 634mg sodium, 125mg potassium

Bacon Beef Strips

Yield: 4 servings | **Prep time:** 15 minutes | **Cook time:** 5 hours

Ingredients:
- 1-pound beef tenderloin, cut into strips
- 4 oz bacon, sliced
- ½ teaspoon ground black pepper
- ½ cup of water

Method:
1. Mix beef with ground black pepper.
2. Then wrap every beef strip with sliced bacon and arrange it in the slow cooker.
3. Add water and close the lid.
4. Cook the meal on High for 5 hours.

Nutritional info per serve: 258 calories, 28.9g protein, 0.4g carbohydrates, 14.8g fat, 0.1g fiber, 90mg cholesterol, 869mg sodium, 379mg potassium.

Beef Curry

Yield: 3 servings | **Prep time:** 10 minutes | **Cook time:** 8 hours

Ingredients:
- 7 oz beef tenderloin, chopped
- 1 teaspoon curry powder
- 1 cup of coconut milk
- ¼ cup of water
- ½ cup cauliflower, chopped
- 1 yellow onion, sliced

Method:
1. Mix coconut milk with curry powder and pour the liquid into the slow cooker.
2. Add beef, cauliflower, and sliced onion.
3. Then add water and close the lid.
4. Cook the meal on low for 8 hours.

Nutritional info per serve: 341 calories, 21.8g protein, 9.1g carbohydrates, 25.3g fat, 3.2g fiber, 61mg cholesterol, 58mg sodium, 561mg potassium.

Cilantro Pork Chops

Yield: 4 servings | **Prep time:** 10 minutes | **Cook time:** 8 hours

Ingredients:
- 4 pork chops
- 1 teaspoon dried cilantro
- 1 teaspoon coconut oil, melted
- 1 teaspoon lemon juice
- ¼ cup of coconut milk

Method:
1. In the shallow bowl mix dried cilantro, olive oil, and lemon juice.
2. Brush the pork chops with cilantro mixture from both sides and transfer in the slow cooker.
3. Add coconut milk and cook on Low for 8 hours.

Nutritional info per serve: 301 calories, 18.3g protein, 0.9g carbohydrates, 24.6g fat, 0.3g fiber, 69mg cholesterol, 349mg sodium, 317mg potassium.

Beef Casserole

Yield: 5 servings | **Prep time:** 10 minutes | **Cook time:** 7 hours

Ingredients:
- 7 oz ground beef
- 1 cup Cheddar cheese, shredded
- ½ cup coconut milk
- 1 teaspoon Italian seasonings
- ½ cup broccoli, chopped

Method:
1. Mix ground beef with Italian seasonings and put it in the slow cooker.
2. Top the meat with broccoli and Cheddar cheese.
3. Then pour the coconut milk over the casserole mixture and close the lid.
4. Cook the casserole on Low for 7 hours.

Nutritional info per serve: 186 calories, 18.1g protein, 1.7g carbohydrates, 11.6g fat, 0.2g fiber, 64mg cholesterol, 178mg sodium, 220mg potassium.

Tender Goulash

Yield: 4 servings | **Prep time:** 10 minutes | **Cook time:** 9 hours

Ingredients:
- 1 onion, chopped
- 1 teaspoon almond flour
- 1 teaspoon ground turmeric
- 1 teaspoon ground
- paprika
- 1-pound pork chunk, chopped
- 1 teaspoon keto tomato paste
- 1 cup of water

Method:
1. Mix water with almond flour until smooth and pour in the slow cooker.
2. Add onion, ground turmeric, paprika, pork chunk, keto tomato paste.
3. Gently stir the goulash mixture and cook it on Low for 9 hours.

Nutritional info per serve: 256 calories, 30.3g protein, 4g carbohydrates, 12.1g fat, 1g fiber, 89mg cholesterol, 924mg sodium, 83mg potassium.

Garlic Pork Ribs

Yield: 3 servings | **Prep time:** 10 minutes | **Cook time:** 5.5 hours

Ingredients:
- 8 oz pork ribs, chopped
- 1 teaspoon garlic powder
- 1 teaspoon coconut oil, melted
- ½ cup of water

Method:
1. Preheat the skillet until hot.
2. Then sprinkle the pork ribs with garlic powder and coconut oil and put them in the hot skillet.
3. Roast the ribs for 3 minutes per side or until they are light brown.
4. Then transfer the pork ribs to the slow cooker.
5. Add water and cook the ribs on high for 5.5 hours.

Nutritional info per serve: 212 calories, 20.2g protein, 0.8g carbohydrates, 13.6g fat, 0.2g fiber, 78mg cholesterol, 433mg sodium, 233mg potassium.

Chayote Squash Pork

Yield: 4 servings | **Prep time:** 10 minutes | **Cook time:** 8 hours

Ingredients:
- 1-pound pork tenderloin, chopped
- 1 teaspoon ground cinnamon
- 1 tablespoon
- Erythritol
- ½ cup Chayote squash, chopped
- 1 cup of water

Method:
1. Mix chayote squash with ground cinnamon and put in the slow cooker.
2. Add water, Erythritol, and pork tenderloin.
3. Close the lid and cook the meal on Low for 8 hours.

Nutritional info per serve: 167 calories, 29.8g protein, 5.1g carbohydrates, 4g fat, 0.4g fiber, 83mg cholesterol, 65mg sodium, 480mg potassium

Cumin Pork

Yield: 6 servings | **Prep time:** 10 minutes | **Cook time:** 5 hours

Ingredients:
- 1-pound pork shoulder, chopped
- 1 teaspoon cumin seeds
- 1 teaspoon garlic
- powder
- 1 teaspoon ground nutmeg
- 2 cup of water

Method:
1. Roast the cumin seeds in the skillet for 2-3 minutes or until the seeds start to smell.
2. Then place them in the slow cooker.
3. Add all remaining ingredients and close the lid.
4. Cook the pork on high for 5 hours.

Nutritional info per serve: 230 calories, 17.8g protein, 1.7g carbohydrates, 16.4g fat, 0.4g fiber, 68mg cholesterol, 449mg sodium, 295mg potassium

Sweet and Sour Pulled Pork

Yield: 4 servings | **Prep time:** 10 minutes | **Cook time:** 6 hours

Ingredients:
- 1-pound pork sirloin
- 2 cups of water
- 2 tablespoons keto ketchup
- 2 tablespoons lemon juice
- 1 teaspoon cayenne pepper
- 1 teaspoon Erythritol

Method:
1. Pour water into the slow cooker.
2. Add pork sirloin and close the lid.
3. Cook the meat on high for 6 hours.
4. Then drain water and shred the meat.
5. Add ketchup, lemon juice, cayenne pepper, and Erythritol.
6. Stir the mixture carefully and transfer to the serving plates.

Nutritional info per serve: 207 calories, 23.3g protein, 3.7g carbohydrates, 10.2g fat, 0.2g fiber, 80mg cholesterol, 154mg sodium, 49mg potassium.

Sandwich Pork Chops

Yield: 2 servings | **Prep time:** 10 minutes | **Cook time:** 4.5 hours

Ingredients:
- 2 pork chops
- 1 teaspoon keto mayonnaise
- 1 teaspoon ground black pepper
- ¼ teaspoon garlic powder
- ½ cup of water

Method:
1. Pour water into the slow cooker.
2. Add garlic powder and ground black pepper.
3. Then add pork chops and cook them on High for 4.5 hours.
4. Remove the cooked pork chops from the water and brush with mayonnaise.

Nutritional info per serve: 269 calories, 18.2g protein, 1.5g carbohydrates, 20.7g fat, 0.3g fiber, 69mg cholesterol, 76mg sodium, 293mg potassium.

Oregano Pork Strips

Yield: 4 servings | **Prep time:** 5 minutes | **Cook time:** 7 hours

Ingredients:
- 12 oz pork tenderloin, cut into strips
- 1 tablespoon dried oregano
- 1 cup of water

Method:
1. Place pork strips in the slow cooker.
2. Add all remaining ingredients and close the lid.
3. Cook the pork strips on Low for 7 hours.
4. Serve the cooked meal with hot gravy from the slow cooker.

Nutritional info per serve: 125 calories, 22.4g protein, 0.7g carbohydrates, 3.1g fat, 0.5g fiber, 62mg cholesterol, 632mg sodium, 378mg potassium

Tomato Pork Sausages

Yield: 5 servings | **Prep time:** 10 minutes | **Cook time:** 7 hours

Ingredients:
- 1-pound pork sausages, chopped, homemade
- 2 tomatoes, chopped
- ½ cup of water
- 1 tablespoon coconut oil
- 1 teaspoon chili powder

Method:
1. Mix pork sausages with chili powder and transfer to the slow cooker.
2. Add coconut oil, water, and tomatoes.
3. Close the lid and cook the meal on Low for 7 hours.

Nutritional info per serve: 342 calories, 18.3g protein, 3.1g carbohydrates, 28.3g fat, 1g fiber, 82mg cholesterol, 1170mg sodium, 448mg potassium

Taco Pork

Yield: 5 servings | **Prep time:** 10 minutes | **Cook time:** 5 hours

Ingredients:
- 1-pound pork shoulder, chopped
- 1 tablespoon taco seasonings
- 1 tablespoon lemon juice
- 1 cup of water
- Method:

1. Mix pork shoulder with taco seasonings and place in the slow cooker.
2. Add water and cook it on High for 5 hours.
3. After this, transfer the cooked meat into the bowl and shred gently with the help of the fork.
4. Add lemon juice and shake gently.

Nutritional info per serve: 274 calories, 21.1g protein, 1.7g carbohydrates, 19.4g fat, 0g fiber, 82mg cholesterol, 232mg sodium, 303mg potassium

Salsa Meat

Yield: 4 servings | **Prep time:** 10 minutes | **Cook time:** 4 hours

Ingredients:
- 1-pound pork sirloin, sliced
- 1 cup keto tomatillo salsa
- 2 garlic cloves, diced
- 1 teaspoon apple cider vinegar
- ½ cup of water

Method:
1. Put all ingredients in the slow cooker and carefully mix.
2. Then close the lid and cook the salsa meat on high for 4 hours.

Nutritional info per serve: 214 calories, 23.8g protein, 2.3g carbohydrates, 11.2g fat, 0.4g fiber, 71mg cholesterol, 169mg sodium, 75mg potassium

BBQ Meatballs

Yield: 4 servings | **Prep time:** 10 minutes | **Cook time:** 7 hours

Ingredients:
- 3 tablespoons keto BBQ sauce
- 10 oz minced pork
- 1 garlic clove, diced
- 1 teaspoon chili powder
- 3 tablespoons water
- 1 teaspoon dried cilantro
- 4 tablespoons avocado oil

Method:
1. In the bowl mix minced pork, garlic, chili powder, water, and dried cilantro.
2. Make the medium size meatballs and arrange them in the slow cooker in one layer.
3. Add avocado oil and close the lid.
4. Cook the meatballs on low for 7 hours.
5. When the meatballs are cooked, brush them gently with BBW sauce.

Nutritional info per serve: 239 calories, 18.7g protein, 4.9g carbohydrates, 16.2g fat, 0.3g fiber, 52mg cholesterol, 760mg sodium, 339mg potassium.

Blackberry Minced Meat

Yield: 5 servings | **Prep time:** 10 minutes | **Cook time:** 6 hours

Ingredients:
- ¼ cup blackberries, mashed
- 1-pound ground pork
- 1 tablespoon coconut oil
- ¼ cup of water
- 1 teaspoon chili powder
- 1 teaspoon dried parsley

Method:
1. Melt coconut oil and pour it into the slow cooker.
2. Add ground pork, chili powder, and dried parsley.
3. Then add water and blackberries. Stir the mixture well.
4. Close the lid and cook the meal on Low for 6 hours.

Nutritional info per serve: 158 calories, 23.9g protein, 1g carbohydrates, 6g fat, 0.6g fiber, 66mg cholesterol, 58mg sodium, 405mg potassium.

Pesto Pork Chops

Yield: 4 servings | **Prep time:** 10 minutes | **Cook time:** 8 hours

Ingredients:
- 4 pork chops
- 4 teaspoons keto pesto sauce
- 4 tablespoons coconut oil

Method:
1. Brush pork chops with pesto sauce.
2. Put coconut oil in the slow cooker.
3. Add pork chops and close the lid.
4. Cook the meat on low for 8 hours.
5. Then transfer the cooked pork chops to the plates and sprinkle with coconut-pesto gravy from the slow cooker.

Nutritional info per serve: 380 calories, 18.6g protein, 0.3g carbohydrates, 33.6g fat, 0.1g fiber, 101mg cholesterol, 89mg sodium, 279mg potassium

Pork Roast with Apples

Yield: 4 servings | **Prep time:** 10 minutes | **Cook time:** 8 hours

Ingredients:
- 1-pound pork shoulder, boneless
- 1 teaspoon Erythritol
- 1 teaspoon allspices
- 1 teaspoon thyme
- 1 apple, chopped
- 1 yellow onion, sliced
- 2 cups of water

Method:
1. Sprinkle the pork shoulder with allspices, thyme, and Erythritol. Transfer it to the slow cooker.
2. Add all remaining ingredients and close the lid.
3. Cook the pork roast on Low for 8 hours.

Nutritional info per serve: 376 calories, 26.9g protein, 11.5g carbohydrates, 24.5g fat, 2.1g fiber, 102mg cholesterol, 83mg sodium, 482mg potassium

Indian Style Cardamom Pork

Yield: 4 servings | **Prep time:** 10 minutes | **Cook time:** 6 hours

Ingredients:

- 1-pound pork steak, tenderized
- 1 teaspoon ground cardamom
- ½ cup of coconut milk
- 1 teaspoon chili powder
- 1 teaspoon ground turmeric
- 1 teaspoon coconut oil
- ¼ cup of water

Method:

1. Cut the pork steak into 4 servings and rub with ground cardamom, chili powder. And ground turmeric.
2. Place the meat in the slow cooker.
3. Add coconut oil, water, and coconut milk.
4. Close the lid and cook the pork on high for 6 hours.

Nutritional info per serve: 295 calories, 21g protein, 7.2g carbohydrates, 21.1g fat, 1.9g fiber, 69mg cholesterol, 569mg sodium, 118mg potassium

Fennel Seeds Pork Chops

Yield: 4 servings | **Prep time:** 10 minutes | **Cook time:** 6 hours

Ingredients:

- 4 pork chops
- 1 tablespoon fennel seeds
- 3 tablespoons avocado oil
- 1 teaspoon garlic, diced
- ½ cup of water

Method:

1. Mix fennel seeds with avocado oil and garlic. Mash the mixture.
2. Then rub the pork chops with fennel seeds mixture and transfer in the slow cooker.
3. Add water and close the lid.
4. Cook the meat on low for 6 hours.

Nutritional info per serve: 276 calories, 18.4g protein, 1.6g carbohydrates, 21.4g fat, 1.1g fiber, 69mg cholesterol, 59mg sodium, 336mg potassium

Pork Rolls

Yield: 2 servings | **Prep time:** 10 minutes | **Cook time:** 4.5 hours

Ingredients:

- 2 pork chops
- 2 oz Mozzarella, sliced
- 1 teaspoon cayenne pepper
- 1 tablespoon keto mayonnaise
- ½ cup of water

Method:

1. Beat the pork chops gently and sprinkle with cayenne pepper.
2. Then brush one side of pork chops with keto mayonnaise and top with mozzarella.
3. Roll the pork chops and secure the prepared rolls with toothpicks.
4. Place the pork rolls in the slow cooker.
5. Add water and cook them on High for 4.5 hours.

Nutritional info per serve: 339 calories, 26.1g protein, 1.5g carbohydrates, 25g fat, 0.2g fiber, 84mg cholesterol, 228mg sodium, 294mg potassium

Braised Ham

Yield: 4 servings | **Prep time:** 10 minutes | **Cook time:** 10 hours

Ingredients:

- 12 oz smoked shoulder ham
- 1 tablespoon mustard
- 2 cups of water
- 1 tablespoon Erythritol

Method:

1. Rub the smoked shoulder ham with mustard and transfer it to the slow cooker.
2. Add water.
3. Close the lid and cook the ham on low for 10 hours.
4. When the time is finished, sprinkle the meat with Erythritol and slice.

Nutritional info per serve: 163 calories, 15.7g protein, 5.8g carbohydrates, 9.8g fat, 0.4g fiber, 50mg cholesterol, 744mg sodium, 20mg potassium

Jamaican Pork Mix

Yield: 4 servings | **Prep time:** 10 minutes | **Cook time:** 4 hours

Ingredients:

- 1 cup of water
- 1 teaspoon Jamaican spices
- 10 oz pork sirloin, chopped
- 1 tomato, chopped
- 1 teaspoon avocado oil

Method:

1. Roast the chopped pork sirloin in avocado oil for 1 minute per side.
2. Then mix the meat with Jamaican spices and transfer in the slow cooker.
3. Add all remaining ingredients and close the lid.
4. Cook the meal on High for 4 hours.

Nutritional info per serve: 174 calories, 23.5g protein, 7.9g carbohydrates, 5.4g fiber, 1.3g fiber, 65mg cholesterol, 629mg sodium, 412mg potassium

Pork Ribs in Soy Sauce

Yield: 5 servings | **Prep time:** 10 minutes | **Cook time:** 5 hours

Ingredients:
- 1-pound pork ribs
- ½ cup of soy sauce
- ½ cup of water
- 1 yellow onion, sliced
- 1 garlic clove, sliced
- ½ teaspoon Erythritol
- ½ teaspoon chili powder

Method:
1. Put all ingredients in the slow cooker and carefully stir them with the help of the spatula.
2. After this, close the lid and cook the pork ribs on high for 5 hours.
3. When the pork ribs are cooked, transfer them to the bowls and top with soy sauce liquid.

Nutritional info per serve: 277 calories, 26.1g protein, 4.9g carbohydrates, 16.4g fat, 0.8g fiber, 93mg cholesterol, 1494mg sodium, 359mg potassium

Apple Cider Vinegar Pulled Pork

Yield: 4 servings | **Prep time:** 15 minutes | **Cook time:** 9 hours

Ingredients:
- ¼ cup apple cider vinegar
- 12 oz pork shoulder
- 1 cup of water
- 1 teaspoon ground black pepper
- 1 teaspoon coconut oil

Method:
1. Put all ingredients in the slow cooker and close the lid.
2. Cook the meat on low for 9 hours.
3. Then open the lid and shred the meat with the help of the forks.

Nutritional info per serve: 272 calories, 19.9g protein, 3.8g carbohydrates, 19.2g fat, 0.2g fiber, 79mg cholesterol, 359mg sodium, 319mg potassium

Sweet Squash Pork

Yield: 4 servings | **Prep time:** 10 minutes | **Cook time:** 4.5 hours

Ingredients:
- ½ cup zucchini, chopped
- 1 tablespoon Erythritol
- 10 oz pork sirloin, sliced
- ½ cup of water
- 1 teaspoon smoked paprika
- ½ teaspoon chili flakes
- 1 teaspoon coconut oil

Method:
1. Melt the coconut oil in the skillet and add sliced pork sirloin.
2. Sprinkle it with smoked paprika and chili flakes and roast for 5 minutes on high heat.
3. Then transfer the meat to the slow cooker, add water, Erythritol, and zucchini.
4. Close the lid and cook the meal on High for 4.5 hours.

Nutritional info per serve: 147 calories, 14.8g protein, 3g carbohydrates, 8g fat, 0.5g fiber, 47mg cholesterol, 46mg sodium, 36mg potassium

Thyme Pork Belly

Yield: 6 servings | **Prep time:** 10 minutes | **Cook time:** 10 hours

Ingredients:
- 10 oz pork belly
- 1 teaspoon ground thyme
- 1 teaspoon ground
- black pepper
- 1 teaspoon garlic powder
- ½ cup of water

Method:
1. In the shallow bowl mix ground thyme, ground black pepper, and garlic powder.
2. Then rub the pork belly with the spice mixture and place it in the slow cooker.
3. Add water and close the lid.
4. Cook the pork belly on Low for 10 hours.
5. Then slice the cooked pork belly into servings.

Nutritional info per serve: 221 calories, 22g protein, 0.7g carbohydrates, 12.7g fat, 0.2g fiber, 55mg cholesterol, 1152mg sodium, 11mg potassium

Beef and Vegetables Stew

Yield: 4 servings | **Prep time:** 10 minutes | **Cook time:** 4 hours

Ingredients:
- 1-pound beef sirloin, chopped
- 1 cup bell pepper, chopped
- 4 cups of water
- 1 tablespoon keto tomato paste
- 1 teaspoon ground coriander
- 1 teaspoon dried sage

Method:
1. Put all ingredients in the slow cooker and close the lid.
2. Cook the stew on Stew mode for 4 hours or according to the directions of your slow cooker.

Nutritional info per serve: 224 calories, 34.8g protein, 3.2g carbohydrates, 7.2g fat, 0.7g fiber, 101mg cholesterol, 85mg sodium, 559mg potassium.

Horseradish Pork Chops

Yield: 4 servings | **Prep time:** 10 minutes | **Cook time:** 5 hours

Ingredients:
- 4 pork chops
- 5 tablespoons horseradish
- ½ cup of water
- 1 onion, sliced
- 1 tablespoon avocado oil

Method:
1. Mix avocado oil with horseradish and rub the pork chops/
2. Put the pork chops and all remaining horseradish mixture in the slow cooker.
3. Add onion and water.
4. Cook the pork chops on high for 5 hours.

Nutritional info per serve: 281 calories, 18.5g protein, 4.9g carbohydrates, 20.5g fat, 1.4g fiber, 69mg cholesterol, 117mg sodium, 373mg potassium

Pork and Cream Cheese Rolls

Yield: 6 servings | **Prep time:** 30 minutes | **Cook time:** 4.5 hours

Ingredients:
- 3 tablespoons cream cheese
- 2 oz bacon, chopped, cooked
- 1-pound pork sirloin
- 1 teaspoon apple cider vinegar
- 1 teaspoon white pepper
- 1 tablespoon avocado oil
- 1 cup of water, for cooking

Method:
1. In the mixing bowl, mix cream cheese with chopped bacon and white pepper.
2. Then slice the pork sirloin into 6 servings.
3. Spread every meat serving with cream cheese mixture and roll.
4. Secure the rolls with the help of the toothpicks if needed.
5. Brush the baking pan with avocado oil and put the meat rolls inside.
6. Pour water into the slow cooker and insert the rack.
7. Place the baking pan with pork rolls on the rack and close the lid.
8. Cook the meal on High for 4.5 hours.

Nutritional info per serve: 219 calories, 27.5g protein, 0.6g carbohydrates, 11g fat, 0.2g fiber, 85mg cholesterol, 276mg sodium, 357mg potassium.

Spaghetti Meatballs

Yield: 4 servings | **Prep time:** 20 minutes | **Cook time:** 3 hours

Ingredients:
- 2 cups ground pork
- 1 teaspoon ground black pepper
- 1 teaspoon dried cilantro
- 1 teaspoon keto tomato paste
- 1 teaspoon coconut oil, melted
- ¼ cup of water

Method:
1. In the mixing bowl mix ground pork with ground black pepper.
2. Then add dried cilantro.
3. Make the small balls from the mixture and press them gently.
4. Pour the coconut oil into the slow cooker.
5. Add water and meatballs.
6. Close the lid and cook the meatballs on high for 3 hours.

Nutritional info per serve: 141 calories, 11.2g protein, 1.6g carbohydrates, 9.8g fat, 0.3g fiber, 42mg cholesterol, 411mg sodium, 231mg potassium

Sweet Pork Tenderloin

Yield: 4 servings | **Prep time:** 35 minutes | **Cook time:** 6 hours

Ingredients:
- 1-pound pork tenderloin
- 1 teaspoon Erythritol
- 1 cup water
- 1 teaspoon cumin seeds
- 1 teaspoon olive oil
- 2 tablespoons soy sauce

Method:
1. Chop the pork tenderloin roughly and put it in the mixing bowl.
2. Add cumin seeds, soy sauce, water, and olive oil. Leave the meat for 30 minutes to marinate.
3. After this, transfer the meat and all liquid to the slow cooker and close the lid.
4. Cook the meat on low for 6 hours.
5. Then remove the meat from the slow cooker and sprinkle it with Erythritol.

Nutritional info per serve: 179 calories, 30.3g protein, 0.8g carbohydrates, 5.3g fat, 0.1g fiber, 83mg cholesterol, 523mg sodium, 514mg potassium

Pork Meatloaf

Yield: 4 servings | **Prep time:** 10 minutes | **Cook time:** 4 hours

Ingredients:

- 8 oz ground pork
- ¼ cup onion, diced
- 1 teaspoon ground black pepper
- 1 teaspoon chili powder
- 1 egg, beaten
- 1 teaspoon olive oil
- 1 teaspoon keto tomato paste
- Cooking spray

Method:

1. Spray the bottom of the slow cooker with cooking spray.

2. After this, mix the ground pork, onion, ground black pepper, chili powder, egg, and olive oil.

3. Transfer the mixture to the slow cooker and flatten it.

4. Then brush the surface of the meatloaf with tomato paste and cook it on High for 4 hours.

Nutritional info per serve: 114 calories, 16.5g protein, 1.7g carbohydrates, 4.4g fat, 0.6g fiber, 82mg cholesterol, 56mg sodium, 297mg potassium

Lemon Stuffed Pork

Yield: 4 servings | **Prep time:** 30 minutes | **Cook time:** 4 hours

Ingredients:

- 1-pound pork loin
- ½ lemon, sliced
- 1 teaspoon dried rosemary
- ½ teaspoon ground paprika
- 2 tablespoons avocado oil

Method:

1. Slice the pork loin into 4 fillets. Beat the pork fillets with the help of the kitchen hammer.

2. After this, rub the meat with dried rosemary and ground pork.

3. Put the lemon slices on the pork fillets and fold them. Secure the meat with toothpicks and brush with avocado oil. Wrap the meat in the foil.

4. Put the wrapped meat in the slow cooker bowl and cook it on Meat mode for 4 hours.

Nutritional info per serve: 288 calories, 31.2g protein, 1.4g carbohydrates, 16.8g fat, 0.7g fiber, 91mg cholesterol, 71mg sodium, 521mg potassium.

Sweet Pork Strips

Yield: 2 servings | **Prep time:** 20 minutes | **Cook time:** 5 hours

Ingredients:

- 6 oz pork loin, cut into strips
- 1 tablespoon Erythritol
- 1 teaspoon ground
- paprika
- 1 teaspoon coconut oil
- 1 cup of water

Method:

1. Pour water into the slow cooker.

2. Add pork strips.

3. Cook the meat on High for 4 hours.

4. Then drain water and transfer the meat to the skillet.

5. Add coconut oil, ground paprika, and roast the meat for 2 minutes per side.

6. Then sprinkle the meat with Erythritol, and carefully mix.

Nutritional info per serve: 252 calories, 23.4g protein, 7.3g carbohydrates, 13.9g fat, 0.4g fiber, 73mg cholesterol, 652mg sodium, 407mg potassium

Cocoa Pork Chops

Yield: 4 servings | **Prep time:** 10 minutes | **Cook time:** 2.5 hours

Ingredients:

- 4 pork chops
- 1 teaspoon cocoa powder
- ½ cup coconut milk
- 1 tablespoon coconut oil
- 1 teaspoon ground black pepper
- ¼ cup of water

Method:

1. Beat the pork chops gently with the help of the kitchen hammer.

2. Then sprinkle the meat with ground black pepper. Transfer it to the slow cooker.

3. After this, mix water with cocoa powder and coconut milk and pour it into the slow cooker.

4. Add coconut oil and close the lid.

5. Cook the pork chops on high for 2.5 hours.

Nutritional info per serve: 305 calories, 18.6g protein, 2g carbohydrates, 24.6g fat, 0.5g fiber, 82mg cholesterol, 378mg sodium, 328mg potassium

Pork and Zucchini Bowl

Yield: 4 servings | **Prep time:** 10 minutes | **Cook time:** 5 hours

Ingredients:

- 12 oz pork stew meat, cubed
- 1 cup zucchini, chopped
- 1 teaspoon white pepper
- 1 teaspoon dried dill
- ½ cup Greek yogurt
- 1 cup of water
- 1 chili pepper, chopped

Method:

1. Put meat in the slow cooker.
2. Add white pepper, dried dill, Greek yogurt, water, and chili pepper.
3. Close the lid and cook the meal on High for 4 hours.
4. Then add zucchini and cook the meal on High for 1 hour more.

Nutritional info per serve: 249 calories, 26.3g protein, 2.8g carbohydrates, 14.3g fat, 0.5g fiber, 86mg cholesterol, 652mg sodium, 452mg potassium

Pork Ragu with Basil

Yield: 4 servings | **Prep time:** 10 minutes | **Cook time:** 4 hours

Ingredients:

- 8 oz pork loin, chopped
- 1 cup rutabaga, peeled, chopped
- 3 oz fennel bulb, chopped
- 1 tablespoon dried
- basil
- 3 cups of water
- ½ cup plain yogurt
- 1 teaspoon keto tomato paste

Method:

1. In the mixing bowl mix keto tomato paste with plain yogurt, dried basil, and pork loin.
2. Transfer the mixture to the slow cooker and close the lid.
3. Cook the meat on high for 2 hours.
4. Then add water and all remaining ingredients. Carefully mix the mixture.
5. Close the lid and cook the ragu on low for 5 hours.

Nutritional info per serve: 178 calories, 17.9g protein, 6.6g carbohydrates, 8.4g fat, 1.6g fiber, 47mg cholesterol, 80mg sodium, 521mg potassium

Apple Cider Vinegar Pork Shoulder

Yield: 4 servings | **Prep time:** 10 minutes | **Cook time:** 10 hours

Ingredients:

- 1-pound pork shoulder, roughly chopped
- 1 cup apple cider vinegar
- 1 cup celery stalk, chopped
- ½ cup yellow onion, chopped
- 1 teaspoon dried thyme
- 1 teaspoon ground paprika

Method:

1. Sprinkle the pork shoulder with dried thyme, and ground paprika.
2. Transfer it to the slow cooker.
3. Add all remaining ingredients and close the lid.
4. Cook the meal on low for 10 hours.

Nutritional info per serve: 392 calories, 26.9g protein, 4.2g carbohydrates, 24.4g fat, 1g fiber, 102mg cholesterol, 683mg sodium, 533mg potassium

White Pepper Pork Cubes

Yield: 2 servings | **Prep time:** 10 minutes | **Cook time:** 4 hours

Ingredients:

- 8 oz pork tenderloin, cubed
- 1 tablespoon keto tomato paste
- 1 tablespoon avocado oil
- 1 teaspoon white pepper

Method:

1. Pour the avocado oil into the skillet and preheat it well.
2. Then put the pork tenderloins in the hot oil and roast on high heat for 3 minutes per side.
3. Transfer the roasted meat to the slow cooker and add all remaining ingredients.
4. Close the lid and cook the pork on high for 4 hours.

Nutritional info per serve: 203 calories, 30.7g protein, 8g carbohydrates, 4.9g fat, 2.3g fiber, 83mg cholesterol, 1274mg sodium, 770mg potassium

Pork Mash

Yield: 4 servings | **Prep time:** 10 minutes | **Cook time:** 4 hours

Ingredients:

- 8 oz ground pork
- 2.5 cups water
- 1 teaspoon chili
- powder
- 1 onion, diced
- 1 teaspoon olive oil

Method:

1. Pour olive oil into the skillet.

2. Add onion and roast the mixture for 4-5 minutes or until the onion is light brown.

3. Transfer it to the slow cooker.

4. Add ground pork and all remaining ingredients.

5. Carefully mix the mixture and cook it on High for 4 hours.

6. Then stir the meal well and transfer it to the serving bowls.

Nutritional info per serve: 104 calories, 15.2g protein, 2.9g carbohydrates, 3.3g fat, 0.8g fiber, 41mg cholesterol, 44mg sodium, 293mg potassium

Pork and Oysters Mushrooms Saute

Yield: 4 servings | **Prep time:** 10 minutes | **Cook time:** 8 hours

Ingredients:

- 1-pound pork tenderloin, chopped
- 6 oz oysters mushrooms, chopped
- 1 cup onion, sliced
- 2 cups of water
- 1 cup coconut milk
- 1 teaspoon ground black pepper

Method:

1. Mix pork tenderloin with ground black pepper and put in the slow cooker.

2. Top the meat with oysters mushrooms and sliced onion.

3. Then add water and coconut milk.

4. Close the lid and cook the meal on low for 8 hours.

Nutritional info per serve: 223 calories, 31.9g protein, 6.3g carbohydrates, 7.5g fat, 1.2g fiber, 94mg cholesterol, 673mg sodium, 685mg potassium

Lemon Pork Belly

Yield: 6 servings | **Prep time:** 10 minutes | **Cook time:** 6 hours

Ingredients:

- 1-pound pork belly
- 2 cups of water
- 1 teaspoon dried thyme
- 1 teaspoon peppercorn
- 2 tablespoons lemon juice

Method:

1. Put all ingredients in the slow cooker and close the lid.

2. Cook the pork belly on High for 6 hours.

3. Then make a quick pressure release and remove the pork belly from the liquid.

4. Slice the pork belly and sprinkle it with lemon liquid from the slow cooker.

Nutritional info per serve: 352 calories, 35g protein, 0.5g carbohydrates, 20.4g fat, 0.2g fiber, 87mg cholesterol, 1225mg sodium, 13mg potassium.

Marinated Pork

Yield: 3 servings | **Prep time:** 20 minutes | **Cook time:** 4 hours

Ingredients:

- 16 oz pork loin, chopped
- ½ cup apple cider vinegar
- 1 tablespoon avocado
- oil
- 1 teaspoon ground coriander
- 1 cup of water

Method:

1. Mix apple cider vinegar with ground coriander.

2. Put the pork loin in the apple cider vinegar liquid and marinate it for 20 minutes.

3. Pour water into the slow cooker.

4. Add avocado oil and meat and close the lid.

5. Cook the meat on High for 4 hours.

Nutritional info per serve: 381 calories, 41.4 protein, 0.6g carbohydrates, 21.6g fat, 0.2g fiber, 121mg cholesterol, 98mg sodium, 685mg potassium.

Pork Ribs Braised in Vinegar

Yield: 4 servings | **Prep time:** 10 minutes | **Cook time:** 6 hours

Ingredients:

- 1-pound pork ribs, roughly chopped
- ½ cup apple cider vinegar
- 2 garlic cloves,
- crushed
- 1 teaspoon Erythritol
- 1 teaspoon clove
- ½ teaspoon chili flakes

Method:

1. Rub the pork ribs with chili flakes and put them in the slow cooker.

2. Add garlic, Erythritol, and clove.

3. Then add the apple cider vinegar, and close the lid.

4. Cook the meal on Low for 6 hours.

Nutritional info per serve: 341 calories, 30.2g protein, 2.4g carbohydrates, 20.2g fat, 0.2g fiber, 117mg cholesterol, 69mg sodium, 369mg potassium

Garlic Pork Loin

Yield: 4 servings | **Prep time:** 15 minutes | **Cook time:** 5 hours

Ingredients:

- 1 teaspoon garlic powder
- 1 garlic clove, diced
- 1-pound pork loin
- 2 tablespoons avocado oil

Method:

1. Rub the pork loin with diced garlic and garlic powder.
2. Then sprinkle the meat with avocado oil and wrap it in the foil.
3. Put the pork in the slow cooker and close the lid.
4. Cook the meal on Meat mode for 5 hours.
5. Then cook the meat till room temperature and transfer it to the serving plates.

Nutritional info per serve: 287 calories, 31.2g protein, 1.2g carbohydrates, 16.7g fat, 0.4g fiber, 91mg cholesterol, 71mg sodium, 513mg potassium.

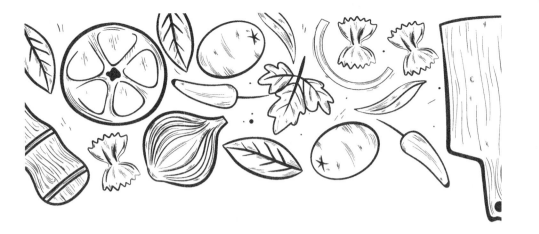

Poultry

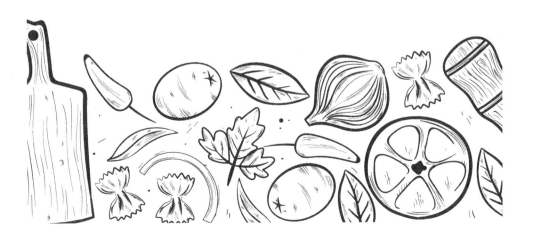

Chives Chicken

Yield: 4 servings | **Prep time:** 10 minutes | **Cook time:** 15 minutes

Ingredients:
- 1-pound chicken fillet, sliced
- 2 oz chives, chopped
- 1 tablespoon coconut oil
- ½ teaspoon onion powder

Method:
1. Sprinkle the chicken fillet with onion powder.
2. Then melt the coconut oil in the slow cooker bowl on saute mode.
3. Add chives.
4. After this, add chicken fillet.
5. Roast the chicken with onion for 10 minutes on saute mode. Stir the chicken from time to time to avoid burning.

Nutritional info per serve: 250 calories, 33.3g protein, 0.9g carbohydrates, 11.9g fat, 0.4g fiber, 101mg cholesterol, 98mg sodium, 320mg potassium.

Tarragon Chicken

Yield: 10 servings | **Prep time:** 5 minutes | **Cook time:** 20 minutes

Ingredients:
- 1-pound chicken breast, skinless, boneless, chopped
- 1 tablespoon dried tarragon
- 1 tablespoon avocado oil

Method:
1. Sprinkle the chicken with dried tarragon and avocado oil.
2. Then put the chicken in the slow cooker and cook it for 10 minutes per side on saute mode.

Nutritional info per serve: 54 calories, 9.7g protein, 0.2g carbohydrates, 1.3g fat, 0.1g fiber, 29mg cholesterol, 23mg sodium, 178mg potassium.

Chicken Pockets

Yield: 4 servings | **Prep time:** 10 minutes | **Cook time:** 4 hours

Ingredients:
- 4 tablespoons plain yogurt
- 1 oz fresh cilantro, chopped
- ½ teaspoon dried thyme
- 1-pound chicken fillet, sliced
- 2 tablespoons cream cheese
- 1 red onion, sliced
- 1/3 cup water
- 4 keto tortillas

Method:
1. Mix plain yogurt with chicken, water, dried thyme, and transfer to the slow cooker.
2. Cook the chicken for 4 hours on High.
3. Then fill the keto tortillas with cream cheese, onion, cilantro, and chicken.

Nutritional info per serve: 407 calories, 46.5g protein, 12.1g carbohydrates, 18.4g fat, 4.8g fiber, 107mg cholesterol, 368mg sodium, 396mg potassium.

Chicken Bowl

Yield: 6 servings | **Prep time:** 15 minutes | **Cook time:** 4 hours

Ingredients:
- 1-pound chicken breast, skinless, boneless, chopped
- 1 teaspoon ground paprika
- 1 teaspoon onion powder
- 1 tomato, chopped
- 1 cup of water
- 1 teaspoon olive oil

Method:
1. Mix chopped chicken breast with ground paprika and onion powder. Transfer it to the slow cooker.
2. Add water. Cook the mixture on High for 4 hours.
3. Then drain the liquid and transfer the mixture to the bowl.
4. Add tomato and olive oil. Mix the meal.

Nutritional info per serve: 122 calories, 17.2g protein, 6.3g carbohydrates, 3g fat, 1.1g fiber, 48mg cholesterol, 45mg sodium, 424mg potassium.

Lemon Chicken

Yield: 6 servings | **Prep time:** 10 minutes | **Cook time:** 20 minutes

Ingredients:
- 6 chicken drumsticks, skinless
- ½ lemon, sliced
- 1 tablespoon butter, softened

Method:
1. Grease the slow cooker bowl with butter.
2. Put the chicken drumsticks in the slow cooker and cook them for 10 minutes per side on Saute mode.

Nutritional info per serve: 96 calories, 12.7g protein, 0.5g carbohydrates, 4.6g fat, 0.1g fiber, 46mg cholesterol, 51mg sodium, 99mg potassium.

Sweet Chicken Breast

Yield: 4 servings | **Prep time:** 20 minutes | **Cook time:** 4 hours

Ingredients:
- 2 yellow onions
- 2 tablespoons Erythritol
- 1 tablespoon coconut oil
- ½ cup of water
- 1-pound chicken breast, skinless, boneless
- 1 teaspoon keto curry paste

Method:
1. Rub the chicken breast with curry paste and transfer it to the slow cooker.
2. Slice the onion and add it to the cooker too.
3. Then add water and close the lid.
4. Cook the chicken breast on High for 4 hours.
5. After this, toss the coconut oil in the skillet.
6. Melt it and add chicken.
7. Sprinkle the chicken with Erythritol and roast for 1 minute per side.
8. Slice the chicken breast.

Nutritional info per serve: 186 calories, 24.7g protein, 12.9g carbohydrates, 6.7g fat, 1.2g fiber, 73mg cholesterol, 126mg sodium, 500mg potassium.

Jerk Chicken

Yield: 4 servings | **Prep time:** 15 minutes | **Cook time:** 7 hours

Ingredients:
- 1 lemon
- 1-pound chicken breast, skinless, boneless
- 1 tablespoon taco seasoning
- 1 teaspoon garlic powder
- 1 teaspoon ground black pepper
- ½ teaspoon minced ginger
- 1 tablespoon soy sauce
- 1 cup of water

Method:
1. Chop the lemon and put it in the blender.
2. Add taco seasoning, garlic powder, ground black pepper, minced ginger, and soy sauce.
3. Blend the mixture until smooth.
4. After this, cut the chicken breast into the servings and rub with the lemon mixture carefully.
5. Transfer the chicken to the slow cooker, add water, and cook on Low for 7 hours.

Nutritional info per serve: 150 calories, 24.7g protein, 4.7g carbohydrates, 2.9g fat, 0.7g fiber, 73mg cholesterol, 496mg sodium, 466mg potassium.

Stuffed Chicken Breast

Yield: 4 servings | **Prep time:** 15 minutes | **Cook time:** 6 hours

Ingredients:
- 1-pound chicken breast, skinless, boneless
- 1 tomato, sliced
- 2 oz mozzarella, sliced
- 1 teaspoon fresh basil
- 1 teaspoon olive oil
- 1 cup of water

Method:
1. Make the horizontal cut in the chicken breast in the shape of the pocket.
2. Then fill it with sliced mozzarella, tomato, and basil.
3. Secure the cut with the help of the toothpicks and sprinkle the chicken with olive oil.
4. Place it in the slow cooker and add water.
5. Cook the chicken on low for 6 hours.

Nutritional info per serve: 182 calories, 28.2g protein, 1.1g carbohydrates, 6.5g fat, 0.2g fiber, 80mg cholesterol, 727mg sodium, 458mg potassium.

Paella

Yield: 6 servings | **Prep time:** 10 minutes | **Cook time:** 4 hours

Ingredients:
- 12 oz chicken fillet, chopped
- 4 oz chorizo, chopped
- ½ cup broccoli rice
- 1 teaspoon garlic, diced
- 2 cups chicken stock
- 1 teaspoon dried cilantro
- 1 teaspoon chili flakes
- Cooking spray

Method:
1. Spray the skillet with cooking spray and put the chorizo inside.
2. Roast the chorizo for 2 minutes per side and transfer to the slow cooker.
3. Then put broccoli rice in the slow cooker.
4. Then add all remaining ingredients and carefully stir the paella mixture.
5. Cook it on High for 4 hours.

Nutritional info per serve: 254 calories, 22.3g protein, 13.1g carbohydrates, 11.7g fat, 0.2g fiber, 67mg cholesterol, 538mg sodium, 238mg potassium.

Asian Style Chicken

Yield: 4 servings | **Prep time:** 10 minutes | **Cook time:** 8 hours

Ingredients:

- 1 teaspoon keto hot sauce
- ¼ cup of soy sauce
- 1 teaspoon avocado oil
- 2 oz scallions, chopped
- 1 tablespoon apple cider vinegar
- 1 teaspoon ground coriander
- 1-pound chicken breast, skinless, boneless, roughly chopped

Method:

1. Put all ingredients in the slow cooker.
2. Close the lid and cook the meal on Low for 8 hours.
3. Then transfer the chicken and a little amount of the chicken liquid to the bowls.

Nutritional info per serve: 166 calories, 25.5g protein, 5.5g carbohydrates, 4.1g fat, 0.6g fiber, 73mg cholesterol, 991mg sodium, 557mg potassium.

Oregano Chicken Breast

Yield: 4 servings | **Prep time:** 10 minutes | **Cook time:** 4 hours

Ingredients:

- 1-pound chicken breast, skinless, boneless, roughly chopped
- 1 tablespoon dried oregano
- 1 bay leaf
- 1 teaspoon peppercorns
- 2 cups of water

Method:

1. Pour water into the slow cooker and add peppercorns and bay leaf.
2. Then sprinkle the chicken with the dried oregano and transfer it to the slow cooker.
3. Close the lid and cook the meal on High for 4 hours.

Nutritional info per serve: 135 calories, 24.2g protein, 1.3g carbohydrates, 3g fat, 0.3g fiber, 73mg cholesterol, 643mg sodium, 448mg potassium.

Chicken Pate

Yield: 6 servings | **Prep time:** 15 minutes | **Cook time:** 8 hours

Ingredients:

- 1-pound chicken liver
- 2 cups of water
- 2 tablespoons coconut oil

Method:

1. Put the chicken liver and water in the slow cooker.
2. Cook the mixture for 8 hours on Low.
3. Then drain water and transfer the mixture to the blender.
4. Add coconut oil.
5. Blend the mixture until smooth.
6. Store the pate in the fridge for up to 7 days.

Nutritional info per serve: 169 calories, 18.6g protein, 1.7g carbohydrates, 9.5g fat, 0.3g fiber, 426mg cholesterol, 454mg sodium, 232mg potassium.

Bacon Chicken

Yield: 4 servings | **Prep time:** 10 minutes | **Cook time:** 7 hours

Ingredients:

- 4 bacon slices, cooked
- 4 chicken drumsticks
- ½ cup of water
- ½ teaspoon ground black pepper

Method:

1. Sprinkle the chicken drumsticks with the ground black pepper.
2. Then wrap every chicken drumstick in the bacon and arrange it in the slow cooker.
3. Add water.
4. Cook the meal on Low for 7 hours.

Nutritional info per serve: 184 calories, 19.8g protein, 1.1g carbohydrates, 10.6g fat, 0.1g fiber, 61mg cholesterol, 1099mg sodium, 237mg potassium.

French-Style Chicken

Yield: 4 servings | **Prep time:** 10 minutes | **Cook time:** 7 hours

Ingredients:

- 1 can keto onion soup
- 4 chicken drumsticks
- ½ cup celery stalk, chopped
- 1 teaspoon dried tarragon
- ¼ cup apple cider vinegar

Method:

1. Put ingredients in the slow cooker and carefully mix them.
2. Then close the lid and cook the chicken on low for 7 hours.

Nutritional info per serve: 127 calories, 15.1g protein, 5.8g carbohydrates, 3.7g fat, 0.7g fiber, 40mg cholesterol, 688mg sodium, 185mg potassium.

Lemon Chicken Thighs

Yield: 4 servings | **Prep time:** 10 minutes | **Cook time:** 7 hours

Ingredients:
- 4 chicken thighs, skinless, boneless
- 1 lemon, sliced
- 1 teaspoon ground black pepper
- ½ teaspoon ground nutmeg
- 1 teaspoon olive oil
- 1 cup of water

Method:
1. Rub the chicken thighs with ground black pepper, nutmeg, and olive oil.
2. Then transfer the chicken to the slow cooker.
3. Add lemon and water.
4. Close the lid and cook the meal on LOW for 7 hours.

Nutritional info per serve: 294 calories, 42.5g protein, 1.8g carbohydrates, 12.2g fat, 0.6g fiber, 130mg cholesterol, 128mg sodium, 383mg potassium.

Chicken Masala

Yield: 4 servings | **Prep time:** 15 / minutes | **Cook time:** 4 hours

Ingredients:
- 1 teaspoon garam masala
- 1 teaspoon ground ginger
- 1 cup of coconut milk
- 1-pound chicken fillet, sliced
- 1 teaspoon olive oil

Method:
1. Mix coconut milk with ground ginger, garam masala, and olive oil.
2. Add chicken fillet and mix the ingredients.
3. Then transfer them to the slow cooker and cook on High for 4 hours.

Nutritional info per serve: 365 calories, 34.2g protein, 3.6g carbohydrates, 23.9g fat, 1.4g fiber, 101mg cholesterol, 108mg sodium, 439mg potassium.

Chicken Minestrone

Yield: 4 servings | **Prep time:** 10 minutes | **Cook time:** 3.5 hours

Ingredients:
- 10 oz chicken fillet, sliced
- 2 cup of water
- 1 teaspoon chili powder
- 1 teaspoon ground paprika
- 1 teaspoon ground cumin
- 1 cup swiss chard, chopped
- 1 cup rutabaga, chopped

Method:
1. Sprinkle the chicken fillet with chili powder, ground paprika, and ground cumin.
2. Transfer it to the slow cooker.
3. Add rutabaga, water, and Swiss chard.
4. Close the lid and cook the meal on High for 3.5 hours.

Nutritional info per serve: 189 calories, 23.9g protein, 10g carbohydrates, 5.8g fat, 2.9g fiber, 63mg cholesterol, 95mg sodium, 505mg potassium.

Vinegar Chicken

Yield: 4 servings | **Prep time:** 15 minutes | **Cook time:** 7 hours

Ingredients:
- 2 tablespoons apple cider vinegar
- 1 cup of water
- 1 teaspoon dried basil
- 1 teaspoon dried oregano
- 1-pound chicken fillet, sliced
- 1 teaspoon mustard

Method:
1. Mix chicken fillet with mustard and apple cider vinegar.
2. Add dried basil, oregano, and transfer to the slow cooker.
3. Add water and close the lid.
4. Cook the chicken on low for 7 hours.

Nutritional info per serve: 222 calories, 33.1g protein, 0.6g carbohydrates, 8.7g fat, 0.3g fiber, 101mg cholesterol, 100mg sodium, 294mg potassium.

Italian Style Chicken

Yield: 4 servings | **Prep time:** 10 minutes | **Cook time:** 6 hours

Ingredients:
- 4 chicken drumsticks, skinless
- 1 teaspoon dried oregano
- ½ teaspoon dried thyme
- 2 tablespoons avocado oil

Method:
1. Rub the chicken drumsticks with thyme and oregano.
2. Then sprinkle the chicken with avocado oil and put it in the slow cooker.
3. Close the lid and cook the chicken on Low for 6 hours.

Nutritional info per serve: 89 calories, 12.8g protein, 0.7g carbohydrates, 3.6g fat, 0.5g fiber, 40mg cholesterol, 37mg sodium, 121mg potassium.

BBQ Chicken

Yield: 2 servings | **Prep time:** 15 minutes | **Cook time:** 7 hours

Ingredients:
- 1 teaspoon minced garlic
- ½ cup keto BBQ sauce
- 1 tablespoon avocado oil
- 3 tablespoons lemon juice
- ½ cup of water
- 7 oz chicken fillet, sliced

Method:
1. In the bowl mix BBQ sauce, minced garlic, avocado oil, and lemon juice.
2. Add chicken fillet and mix the mixture.
3. After this, transfer it to the slow cooker. Add water and close the lid.
4. Cook the chicken on low for 7 hours.

Nutritional info per serve: 217 calories, 29.1g protein, 4.1g carbohydrates, 8.7g fat, 0.4g fiber, 88mg cholesterol, 241mg sodium, 298mg potassium.

Keto Sweet Chicken

Yield: 6 servings | **Prep time:** 10 minutes | **Cook time:** 6 hours

Ingredients:
- 1 teaspoon chili flakes
- 6 chicken drumsticks
- 2 tablespoons Erythritol
- 1 tablespoon coconut
- oil, melted
- 1 tablespoon lemon juice
- 1 teaspoon ground black pepper
- ¼ cup coconut milk

Method:
1. In the bowl mix chili flakes, Erythritol, coconut oil, lemon juice, and ground black pepper.
2. Then brush every chicken drumstick with the sweet mixture and transfer it to the slow cooker.
3. Add coconut milk and close the lid. Cook the meal on Low for 6 hours.

Nutritional info per serve: 113 calories, 13.1g protein, 3.7g carbohydrates, 4.8g fat, 0.1g fiber, 46mg cholesterol, 57mg sodium, 110mg potassium.

Chili Drumsticks

Yield: 4 servings | **Prep time:** 10 minutes | **Cook time:** 30 minutes

Ingredients:
- 4 chicken drumsticks, skinless
- 1 teaspoon chili flakes
- 1 teaspoon dried sage
- 1 tablespoon avocado oil

Method:
1. In the shallow bowl, mix chili flakes, and dried sage.
2. Then mix chicken drumsticks with spice mixture.
3. After this, preheat the slow cooker on Saute mode for 3-4 minutes.
4. Put the chicken drumsticks in the hot slow cooker bowl and roast the meal for 10 minutes per side on the saute mode.

Nutritional info per serve: 83 calories, 12.7g protein, 0.3g carbohydrates, 3.1g fat, 0.2g fiber, 40mg cholesterol, 37mg sodium, 105mg potassium.

Provence Style Chicken Cubes

Yield: 4 servings | **Prep time:** 10 minutes | **Cook time:** 4 hours

Ingredients:
- 1 teaspoon herb de Provence
- 1 teaspoon Erythritol
- 1 tablespoon keto BBQ sauce
- 1 yellow onion, diced
- 1 teaspoon garlic powder
- 1-pound chicken fillet, cubed
- 1 cup of water

Method:
1. Put all ingredients in the slow cooker.
2. Mix the ingredients until homogenous.
3. Then close the lid and cook the meal on high for 4 hours.

Nutritional info per serve: 304 calories, 33.2g protein, 5.9g carbohydrates, 8.5g fat, 0.7g fiber, 101mg cholesterol, 143mg sodium, 333mg potassium.

Garlic and Dill Chicken

Yield: 4 servings | **Prep time:** 10 minutes | **Cook time:** 3 hours

Ingredients:
- 2 tablespoons avocado oil
- 1 teaspoon minced garlic
- 1 teaspoon dried dill
- 1-pound chicken breast, skinless, boneless

Method:
1. Mix dill with avocado oil and dried dill.
2. Then rub the chicken breast with avocado oil mixture and wrap it in the foil.
3. Put the chicken in the slow cooker and close the lid.
4. Cook the chicken on Saute mode for 3 hours.

Nutritional info per serve: 140 calories, 24.2g protein, 0.8g carbohydrates, 3.7g fat, 0.4g fiber, 73mg cholesterol, 59mg sodium, 453mg potassium.

Orange Chicken

Yield: 4 servings | **Prep time:** 10 minutes | **Cook time:** 8 hours

Ingredients:
- 1 orange, chopped
- 1 teaspoon ground turmeric
- 1 teaspoon peppercorn
- 1 teaspoon olive oil
- 1 cup of water
- 1-pound chicken breast, skinless, boneless, sliced

Method:
1. Put all ingredients in the slow cooker and gently mix them.
2. Close the lid and cook the meal on Low for 8 hours.
3. When the time is finished, transfer the chicken to the serving bowls and top with orange liquid from the slow cooker.

Nutritional info per serve: 164 calories, 24.6g protein, 6.1g carbohydrates, 4.1g fat, 1.g4 fiber, 73mg cholesterol, 641mg sodium, 524mg potassium.

Chili Chicken

Yield: 4 servings | **Prep time:** 15 minutes | **Cook time:** 7 hours

Ingredients:
- 1 teaspoon chili powder
- 1 tablespoon keto hot sauce
- 1 tablespoon coconut oil, melted
- ½ teaspoon ground
- turmeric
- 1 teaspoon garlic, minced
- ½ cup of water
- 1-pound chicken wings

Method:
1. Rub the chicken wings with hot sauce, chili powder, ground turmeric, garlic, and coconut oil.
2. Then pour water into the slow cooker and add prepared chicken wings.
3. Cook the chicken on low for 7 hours.

Nutritional info per serve: 249 calories, 33g protein, 0.8g carbohydrates, 12g fat, 0.3g fiber, 101mg cholesterol, 200mg sodium, 303mg potassium.

Chicken Teriyaki

Yield: 4 servings | **Prep time:** 10 minutes | **Cook time:** 4 hours

Ingredients:
- 1-pound chicken wings
- ½ cup keto teriyaki sauce
- ½ cup of water
- 1 onion, chopped
- 1 teaspoon coconut oil

Method:
1. Toss the coconut oil into the pan and melt it.
2. Add onion and roast the vegetables for 5 minutes on medium heat.
3. Then transfer them to the slow cooker.
4. Add chicken wings, keto teriyaki sauce, and water.
5. Close the lid and cook the meal for 4 hours on High.

Nutritional info per serve: 273 calories, 35.4g protein, 9.7g carbohydrates, 9.4g fat, 1g fiber, 103mg cholesterol, 1497mg sodium, 446mg potassium.

Thyme Whole Chicken

Yield: 6 servings | **Prep time:** 15 minutes | **Cook time:** 9 hours

Ingredients:
- 1.5-pound whole chicken
- 1 tablespoon dried
- thyme
- 1 tablespoon olive oil
- 1 cup of water

Method:
1. Chop the whole chicken roughly and sprinkle with dried thyme and olive oil.
2. Then transfer it to the slow cooker, add water.
3. Cook the chicken on low for 9 hours.

Nutritional info per serve: 237 calories, 32.9g protein, 0.3g carbohydrates, 10.8g fat, 0.2g fiber, 101mg cholesterol, 487mg sodium, 280mg potassium.

Thai Chicken

Yield: 4 servings | **Prep time:** 15 minutes | **Cook time:** 4 hours

Ingredients:
- 12 oz chicken fillet, sliced
- ½ cup of coconut milk
- 1 teaspoon dried lemongrass
- 1 teaspoon chili
- powder
- 1 teaspoon keto tomato paste
- 1 teaspoon ground cardamom
- 1 cup of water

Method:
1. Rub the chicken with chili powder, tomato paste, ground cardamom, and dried lemongrass. Transfer it to the slow cooker.
2. Add water and coconut milk.
3. Close the lid and cook the meal on High for 4 hours.

Nutritional info per serve: 236 calories, 25.5g protein, 2.7g carbohydrates, 13.6g fat, 1.1g fiber, 76mg cholesterol, 87mg sodium, 321mg potassium.

Mexican Chicken

Yield: 2 servings | **Prep time:** 10 minutes | **Cook time:** 6 hours

Ingredients:

- ½ cup bell pepper, sliced
- 1 teaspoon cayenne pepper
- 2 chicken thighs,
- skinless, boneless
- 1 yellow onion, sliced
- ½ cup keto Salsa Verde
- 1 cup of water

Method:

1. Pour water into the slow cooker.
2. Add salsa Verde and onion.
3. Then add cayenne pepper and chicken thighs.
4. Cook the mixture on High for 3 hours.
5. After this, add bell pepper and cook the meal on Low for 3 hours.

Nutritional info per serve: 327 calories, 44g protein, 10.5g carbohydrates, 11.3g fat, 2.1g fiber, 130mg cholesterol, 477mg sodium, 510mg potassium.

Easy Chicken Adobo

Yield: 4 servings | **Prep time:** 10 minutes | **Cook time:** 4 hours

Ingredients:

- 1 teaspoon minced garlic
- 1 yellow onion, chopped
- ½ teaspoon ground ginger
- 4 chicken thighs, skinless, boneless
- 1 tablespoon apple cider vinegar
- 1 tablespoon soy sauce
- ½ teaspoon ground black pepper
- ½ cup of water

Method:

1. Put the onion in the slow cooker.
2. Then mix soy sauce with apple cider vinegar and minced garlic.
3. Rub the chicken with garlic mixture and put it in the slow cooker.
4. Then add ground black pepper, ginger, and water.
5. Cook the meal on High for 4 hours.

Nutritional info per serve: 294 calories, 42.9g protein, 3.6g carbohydrates, 10.9g fat, 0.8g fiber, 130g cholesterol, 354mg sodium, 418mg potassium.

Fennel and Chicken Saute

Yield: 4 servings | **Prep time:** 10 minutes | **Cook time:** 7 hours

Ingredients:

- 1 cup fennel, peeled, chopped
- 10 oz chicken fillet, chopped
- 1 tablespoon keto tomato paste
- 1 cup of water
- 1 teaspoon ground black pepper
- 1 teaspoon olive oil
- ½ teaspoon fennel seeds

Method:

1. Heat the olive oil in the skillet.
2. Add fennel seeds and roast them until you get a saturated fennel smell.
3. Transfer the seeds to the slow cooker.
4. Add fennel, chicken fillet, tomato paste, water, and ground black pepper.
5. Close the lid and cook the meal on Low for 7 hours.

Nutritional info per serve: 157 calories, 28.1g protein, 2.8g carbohydrates, 6.5g fat, 1.1g fiber, 63mg cholesterol, 78mg sodium, 314mg potassium.

Russian Chicken

Yield: 4 servings | **Prep time:** 10 minutes | **Cook time:** 4 hours

Ingredients:

- 2 tablespoons keto mayonnaise
- 4 chicken thighs, skinless, boneless
- 1 teaspoon minced garlic
- 1 teaspoon ground black pepper
- 1 teaspoon avocado oil
- ½ cup of water

Method:

1. In the bowl mix keto mayonnaise, minced garlic, ground black pepper, and oil.
2. Then add chicken thighs and mix the ingredients well.
3. After this, pour water into the slow cooker. Add chicken thighs mixture.
4. Cook the meal on High for 4 hours.

Nutritional info per serve: 319 calories, 42.4g protein, 2.3g carbohydrates, 14.5g fat, 0.2g fiber, 132mg cholesterol, 760mg sodium, 365mg potassium.

Creamy Cocoa Chicken

Yield: 8 servings | **Prep time:** 10 minutes | **Cook time:** 8 hours

Ingredients:
- 2 teaspoons cocoa powder
- 1 cup of water
- 2-pound chicken breast, skinless, boneless
- 1 tablespoon keto tomato paste
- 1 teaspoon keto hot sauce
- ½ cup coconut cream

Method:
1. Whisk cocoa powder with coconut cream until smooth and pour the liquid into the slow cooker.
2. Mix chicken breast with tomato paste and hot sauce and put in the slow cooker.
3. Then add water and close the lid.
4. Cook the chicken on low for 8 hours.
5. Then shred the chicken and serve it with cocoa gravy.

Nutritional info per serve: 144 calories, 24.5g protein, 1.6g carbohydrates, 3.9g fat, 0.5g fiber, 75mg cholesterol, 82mg sodium, 480mg potassium.

Coconut Chicken

Yield: 6 servings | **Prep time:** 10 minutes | **Cook time:** 40 minutes

Ingredients:
- 1-pound chicken breast, skinless, boneless, chopped
- ½ cup coconut cream
- 1 teaspoon dried oregano
- 1 teaspoon garlic powder
- ½ teaspoon ground paprika
- 1 tablespoon coconut oil

Method:
1. In the shallow bowl, mix ground paprika, garlic powder, and dried oregano.
2. Then mix the chicken breast with ground paprika mixture.
3. Then melt the coconut oil in the slow cooker bowl on saute mode.
4. Add chicken and roast it for 4 minutes per side on saute mode.
5. Add coconut cream and close the lid.
6. Cook the meal on high (manual mode) for 30 minutes.

Nutritional info per serve: 155 calories, 16.6g protein, 1.7g carbohydrates, 9g fat, 0.7g fiber, 48mg cholesterol, 42mg sodium, 346mg potassium.

Curry Chicken Wings

Yield: 4 servings | **Prep time:** 15 minutes | **Cook time:** 7 hours

Ingredients:
- 1-pound chicken wings
- 1 teaspoon curry paste
- ½ cup coconut cream
- 1 teaspoon minced garlic
- ½ teaspoon ground nutmeg
- ½ cup of water

Method:
1. In the bowl mix curry paste, coconut cream, minced garlic, and ground nutmeg.
2. Add chicken wings and stir.
3. Then pour water into the slow cooker.
4. Add chicken wings with all remaining curry paste mixture and close the lid.

Cook the chicken wings on Low for 7 hours.

Nutritional info per serve: 278 calories, 33.2g protein, 1.1g carbohydrates, 14.8g fat, 0.1g fiber, 121mg cholesterol, 104mg sodium, 291mg potassium.

Cheese Chicken Casserole

Yield: 6 servings | **Prep time:** 15 minutes | **Cook time:** 4 hours

Ingredients:
- 1-pound chicken breast, skinless, boneless, chopped
- 1 cup Cheddar cheese, shredded
- 1 tablespoon coconut oil, softened
- ½ teaspoon chili flakes
- ½ cup of water
- 1 cup bell pepper, chopped
- 1 cup water, for cooking

Method:
1. Grease the slow cooker casserole mold with coconut oil.
2. Then mix chicken breast with chili flakes and put in the casserole mold in one layer.
3. Top it with bell pepper and water.
4. Then add Cheddar cheese and flatten it well.
5. Pour the 1 cup of water into the slow cooker and insert the rack.
6. Put the casserole mold on the rack and close the lid.
7. Cook the meal on manual (high pressure) for 4 hours.

Nutritional info per serve: 288 calories, 20.9g protein, 1.8g carbohydrates, 10.5g fat, 0.3g fiber, 68mg cholesterol, 157mg sodium, 336mg potassium.

Stuffed Whole Chicken

Yield: 10 servings | **Prep time:** 15 minutes | **Cook time:** 6 hours

Ingredients:

- 3-pound whole chicken
- 1 tablespoon taco seasonings
- 1 lemon, sliced
- 1 tablespoon olive oil
- 2 cups of water

Method:

1. Fill the chicken with sliced lemon.
2. Then rub the chicken with taco seasonings and brush with olive oil.
3. Place it in the slow cooker. Add water.
4. Cook the chicken on High for 6 hours.
5. When the chicken is cooked, chop it into servings and serve with cooked lemon slices.

Nutritional info per serve: 285 calories, 39.4g protein, 3.7g carbohydrates, 11.5g fat, 0.5g fiber, 121mg cholesterol, 182mg sodium, 355mg potassium.

Garlic Chicken

Yield: 2 servings | **Prep time:** 10 minutes | **Cook time:** 30 minutes

Ingredients:

- ½ cup almond flour
- 1 egg, beaten
- 2 tablespoons minced garlic
- 2 chicken breasts, skinless, boneless, chopped
- 2 tablespoons coconut oil

Method:

1. Melt the coconut oil in the slow cooker bowl on Saute mode.
2. Then mix chicken with minced garlic and egg.
3. After this, coat the chicken in the almond flour and put in the melted oil.
4. Close the lid and cook the chicken on Manual mode for 30 minutes.

Nutritional info per serve: 479 calories, 47g protein, 4.5g carbohydrates, 30.2g fat, 0.9g fiber, 212mg cholesterol, 160mg sodium, 418mg potassium.

Sage Chicken Wings

Yield: 6 servings | **Prep time:** 10 minutes | **Cook time:** 25 minutes

Ingredients:

- 1 teaspoon dried sage
- 1 teaspoon ground black pepper
- 6 chicken wings,
- skinless
- 1 tablespoon avocado oil

Method:

1. Mix the chicken wings with ground black pepper and dried sage.
2. Then sprinkle the chicken wings with avocado oil and transfer them to the slow cooker.
3. Close the lid and cook the chicken on Saute mode for 10 minutes.
4. Then open the lid and flip the chicken wings on another side. Cook the meal for 10 minutes more.

Nutritional info per serve: 282 calories, 42.3g protein, 0.4g carbohydrates, 11.1g fat, 0.2g fiber, 130mg cholesterol, 126mg sodium, 368mg potassium.

Oregano Chicken Wings

Yield: 2 servings | **Prep time:** 10 minutes | **Cook time:** 20 minutes

Ingredients:

- 4 chicken wings, skinless
- 1 tablespoon dried oregano
- 2 tablespoons avocado oil
- 1 tablespoon lemon juice

Method:

1. Sprinkle the chicken wings with dried oregano, avocado oil, and lemon juice.
2. Then put them in the slow cooker and flatten them in one layer (if possible). Close the lid and cook the chicken wings on saute mode for 10 minutes per one side.

Nutritional info per serve: 305 calories, 42.7g protein, 2.4g carbohydrates, 12.9g fat, 1.6g fiber, 130mg cholesterol, 128mg sodium, 446mg potassium.

Paprika Chicken Wings

Yield: 4 servings | **Prep time:** 10 minutes | **Cook time:** 35 minutes

Ingredients:

- 10 oz chicken wings, skinless
- 1 tablespoon ground paprika
- 1 tablespoon avocado oil
- ½ cup water

Method:

1. Sprinkle the chicken wings with ground paprika.
2. Then sprinkle the chicken wings with avocado oil and put them in the slow cooker.
3. Add water and close the lid.
4. Cook the meal on saute mode for 30 minutes.

Nutritional info per serve: 144 calories, 20.8g protein, 1.2g carbohydrates, 5.9g fat, 0.8g fiber, 63mg cholesterol, 63mg sodium, 224mg potassium.

Chicken Meatballs

Yield: 3 servings | **Prep time:** 10 minutes | **Cook time:** 20 minutes

Ingredients:
- 1 teaspoon dried oregano
- 1 teaspoon chili powder
- 1 teaspoon dried cilantro
- 1 cup ground chicken
- 1 teaspoon coconut oil

Method:
1. In the mixing bowl, mix ground chicken, dried cilantro, chili powder, and dried oregano.
2. Then make the small meatballs.
3. Melt the coconut oil in a slow cooker bowl on saute mode.
4. Then put the chicken meatballs in the hot coconut oil and cook them on saute mode for 4 minutes per side.

Nutritional info per serve: 106 calories, 13.7g protein, 0.8g carbohydrates, 5.2g fat, 0.5g fiber, 42mg cholesterol, 49mg sodium, 139mg potassium.

Lime Chicken Wings

Yield: 5 servings | **Prep time:** 10 minutes | **Cook time:** 30 minutes

Ingredients:
- 5 chicken wings, skinless
- 1 teaspoon lime zest, grated
- 1 tablespoon avocado oil
- 3 tablespoons lime juice
- ½ cup of water

Method:
1. Mix lime juice, avocado oil, and lime zest.
2. Then rub the chicken wings with an avocado oil mixture.
3. Put the chicken wings and water in the slow cooker and close the lid.
4. Cook the chicken wings on manual mode (Saute) for 30 minutes.

Nutritional info per serve: 110 calories, 16.2g protein, 0.2g carbohydrates, 4.5g fat, 0.2g fiber, 50mg cholesterol, 49mg sodium, 146mg potassium.

Almond Chicken

Yield: 4 servings | **Prep time:** 10 minutes | **Cook time:** 1 hour

Ingredients:
- 11 oz chicken fillet
- 2 eggs, beaten
- ½ cup almond flour
- ½ cup organic almond milk

Method:
1. Cut the chicken into 4 servings.
2. Then dip the chicken in the eggs and coat in the almond flour.
3. Pour the almond milk into the slow cooker and add chicken pieces.
4. Close the lid and cook the chicken on high for 1 hour.

Nutritional info per serve: 269 calories, 26.8g protein, 2.6g carbohydrates, 16.9g fat, 1g fiber, 151mg cholesterol, 104mg sodium, 298mg potassium.

Paprika Chicken Fillet

Yield: 5 servings | **Prep time:** 10 minutes | **Cook time:** 20 minutes

Ingredients:
- 1 tablespoon coconut oil
- 1 teaspoon ground paprika
- ½ teaspoon ground turmeric
- 1-pound chicken fillet
- ½ teaspoon keto tomato paste

Method:
1. Put the coconut oil in the slow cooker and melt it on saute mode.
2. Meanwhile, slice the chicken fillet and mix it with ground paprika, ground turmeric, and keto tomato paste.
3. Add the chicken to the coconut oil and saute it for 7 minutes per side.

Nutritional info per serve: 198 calories, 26.3g protein, 0.4g carbohydrates, 9.5g fat, 0.2g fiber, 81mg cholesterol, 78mg sodium, 236mg potassium.

Lemon Duck Breast

Yield: 4 servings | **Prep time:** 10 minutes | **Cook time:** 4 hours

Ingredients:
- 1-pound duck breast, skinless, boneless, chopped
- 1 lemon, sliced
- 1 tablespoon olive oil
- 1 cup of water

Method:
1. Sprinkle the duck fillet with olive oil and put it in the slow cooker.
2. Top it with sliced lemon and roast on saute mode for 5 minutes per side.
3. Then add water and close the lid.
4. Cook the duck breast on High for 4 hours.

Nutritional info per serve: 181 calories, 25.1g protein, 1.4g carbohydrates, 8.1g fat, 0.4g fiber, 0mg cholesterol, 2mg sodium, 21mg potassium.

Cheddar Chicken Thighs

Yield: 4 servings | **Prep time:** 10 minutes | **Cook time:** 5 hours

Ingredients:

- 4 chicken thighs, boneless, skinless
- 5 oz Cheddar cheese, shredded
- 1 tablespoon coconut oil
- 1 teaspoon dried cilantro
- ½ teaspoon cayenne pepper

Method:

1. Mix chicken thighs with dried cilantro and cayenne pepper.
2. Put it in the slow cooker bowl.
3. Add coconut oil and shredded cheese.
4. Close the lid and cook the chicken on Low for 5 hours.

Nutritional info per serve: 450 calories, 51.1g protein, 0.6g carbohydrates, 26g fat, 0.1g fiber, 167mg cholesterol, 346mg sodium, 395mg potassium.

Chicken Pie

Yield: 6 servings | **Prep time:** 10 minutes | **Cook time:** 7 hours

Ingredients:

- 1 cup coconut flour
- 2 tablespoons butter, softened
- ½ teaspoon ground black pepper
- 1 egg, beaten
- 1 cup ground chicken
- 1 teaspoon dried dill
- 1 oz Cheddar cheese, shredded
- 1 cup of water, for cooking

Method:

1. In the mixing bowl, mix coconut flour with butter. Knead the dough.
2. Then put the dough in the slow cooker baking pan and flatten it in the shape of the pie crust.
3. After this, mix ground black pepper with ground chicken, dill, and Cheddar cheese.
4. Put the ground chicken over the pie crust, flatten it well.
5. Then pour the beaten egg over the ground chicken.
6. Pour water into the slow cooker bowl and insert the rack.
7. Place the pie on the rack and close the lid.
8. Cook it for 7 hours on low.

Nutritional info per serve: 202 calories, 12.9g protein, 12.3g carbohydrates, 12.6g fat, 6.7g fiber, 63mg cholesterol, 107mg sodium, 80mg potassium.

Masala Chicken Thighs

Yield: 3 servings | **Prep time:** 15 minutes | **Cook time:** 40 minutes

Ingredients:

- 3 chicken thighs, boneless, skinless
- ¼ cup coconut cream
- 1 teaspoon garam masala
- ½ teaspoon dried thyme
- 1 tablespoon avocado oil

Method:

1. In the mixing bowl, mix garam masala, coconut cream, and dried thyme.
2. Then preheat the avocado oil in the slow cooker for 2 minutes on saute mode and add chicken thighs.
3. Roast them for 3 minutes per side.
4. Add coconut cream mixture and close the lid.
5. Simmer the chicken thighs for 30 minutes on saute mode.

Nutritional info per serve: 330 calories, 42.8g protein, 1.5g carbohydrates, 16.2g fat, 0.7g fiber, 130mg cholesterol, 130mg sodium, 424mg potassium.

Duck with Zucchinis

Yield: 2 servings | **Prep time:** 10 minutes | **Cook time:** 4 hours

Ingredients:

- 10 oz duck breast, skinless, boneless
- 1 zucchini, sliced
- 1 teaspoon ground black pepper
- 1 tablespoon avocado oil
- 1 teaspoon keto tomato paste
- 1 teaspoon cayenne pepper
- 1 cup of water

Method:

1. Mix keto tomato paste with avocado oil, cayenne pepper, and ground black pepper. Add water and whisk well.
2. Then mix duck breast with tomato mixture and transfer in the slow cooker.
3. Add zucchini.
4. Close the lid and cook the meal on High for 4 hours.

Nutritional info per serve: 216 calories, 32.8g protein, 5.4g carbohydrates, 6.9g fat, 2.1g fiber, 0mg cholesterol, 16mg sodium, 339mg potassium.

Chicken with Olives

Yield: 2 servings | **Prep time:** 10 minutes | **Cook time:** 5 hours

Ingredients:

- 2 kalamata olives, pitted, sliced
- 2 chicken thighs, skinless, boneless
- 1 teaspoon chili powder
- 1 tablespoon lemon juice
- 1 tablespoon avocado oil

Method:

1. Brush the slow cooker bowl with avocado oil.
2. Then mix the chicken thighs with chili powder and lemon juice.
3. Put the chicken inside the slow cooker bowl.
4. Top the chicken with Kalamata olives and cover with foil.
5. Cook the meal on low for 5 hours.

Nutritional info per serve: 298 calories, 42.6g protein, 1.5g carbohydrates, 12.5g fat, 0.9g fiber, 130mg cholesterol, 179mg sodium, 412mg potassium.

Turkey Bake

Yield: 6 servings | **Prep time:** 10 minutes | **Cook time:** 7 hours

Ingredients:

- 1-pound turkey breast, skinless, boneless, chopped
- ½ cup Cheddar cheese, shredded
- 2 zucchinis, chopped
- 1 teaspoon chili powder
- 1 teaspoon white pepper
- ½ teaspoon dried sage
- 1 tablespoon coconut oil
- 1 teaspoon avocado oil
- ½ cup coconut cream

Method:

1. Mix the turkey breast with chili powder, white pepper, dried sage, and avocado oil.
2. Then put the turkey breast in the slow cooker.
3. Top the turkey breast with zucchinis, avocado oil, coconut cream, and shredded cheese.
4. Close the lid and cook the turkey on Low for 7 hours.

Nutritional info per serve: 196 calories, 16.6g protein, 7.2g carbohydrates, 11.7g fat, 1.8g fiber, 42mg cholesterol, 840mg sodium, 477mg potassium.

Chicken with Peppers

Yield: 4 servings | **Prep time:** 10 minutes | **Cook time:** 4 hours

Ingredients:

- 12 oz chicken fillet, chopped
- 1 cup bell pepper, roughly chopped
- 1 teaspoon keto tomato paste
- 1 tablespoon coconut oil
- ¼ cup of water
- 1 teaspoon ground black pepper

Method:

1. Mix the chicken fillet with keto tomato paste, ground black pepper, and water and put it in the slow cooker.
2. Add coconut oil and bell peppers.
3. Cook the meal on high for 4 hours.

Nutritional info per serve: 203 calories, 25g protein, 2.9g carbohydrates, 9.8g fat, 0.6g fiber, 76mg cholesterol, 75mg sodium, 283mg potassium.

Parsley Chicken

Yield: 4 servings | **Prep time:** 10 minutes | **Cook time:** 6 hours

Ingredients:

- 1 tablespoon dried parsley
- 1-pound chicken breast, skinless, boneless, chopped
- 1 tablespoon avocado oil

Method:

1. Mix the chicken with dried parsley and avocado oil.
2. Wrap the chicken breast in the foil and put it in the slow cooker.
3. Close the lid and cook the chicken on Low for 6 hours.

Nutritional info per serve: 134 calories, 24.1g protein, 0.3g carbohydrates, 3.3g fat, 0.2g fiber, 73mg cholesterol, 59mg sodium, 436mg potassium.

Coconut Chicken Fillets

Yield: 2 servings | **Prep time:** 10 minutes | **Cook time:** 4 hours

Ingredients:

- 12 oz chicken fillets
- ½ cup coconut cream
- 1 teaspoon ground black pepper
- 1 tablespoon coconut flour
- 1 oz Parmesan, grated
- 1 teaspoon avocado oil

Method:

1. Mix the chicken fillets with ground black pepper and put them in the slow cooker bowl.

2. Add avocado oil and roast the chicken for 4 minutes on saute mode.

3. Add coconut flour and coconut cream and carefully mix the mixture.

4. Then top it with grated Parmesan and close the lid.

5. Cook the chicken on Low for 4 hours.

Nutritional info per serve: 530 calories, 56g protein, 6.9g carbohydrates, 30.9g fat, 3.2g fiber, 162mg cholesterol, 295mg sodium, 592mg potassium.

Oregano Meatballs

Yield: 6 servings | **Prep time:** 10 minutes | **Cook time:** 10 minutes

Ingredients:

- 2 cups ground chicken
- 1 tablespoon dried oregano
- 1 teaspoon ground paprika
- 1 teaspoon garlic powder
- 1 tablespoon avocado oil

Method:

1. In the mixing bowl mix ground chicken with dried oregano, ground paprika, and garlic powder.

2. Then make the medium-size meatballs.

3. Preheat the avocado oil for 2 minutes in the slow cooker. Use saute mode.

4. Put the meatballs in the hot oil and roast for 3 minutes per side on saute mode.

Nutritional info per serve: 97 calories, 13.7g protein, 1.2g carbohydrates, 3.9g fat, 0.6g fiber, 42mg cholesterol, 41mg sodium, 147mg potassium.

Duck Salad

Yield: 4 servings | **Prep time:** 10 minutes | **Cook time:** 16 hours

Ingredients:

- 8 oz duck fillet
- 1 teaspoon mustard
- 1 teaspoon avocado oil
- 1 teaspoon chili powder
- 2 cups lettuce, chopped
- 2 oz Feta, crumbled
- 1 tablespoon olive oil

Method:

1. Mix the duck fillet with avocado oil and mustard and roast in the slow cooker on saute mode for 6 minutes per side.

2. Then slice the duck fillet and put it in the salad bowl.

3. Add chili powder, lettuce, and olive oil.

4. Shake the salad well and top with crumbled feta.

Nutritional info per serve: 149 calories, 19.2g protein, 2.1g carbohydrates, 7.4g fat, 0.6g fiber, 13mg cholesterol, 251mg sodium, 105mg potassium.

Clove Chicken

Yield: 4 servings | **Prep time:** 10 minutes | **Cook time:** 20 minutes

Ingredients:

- 4 chicken thighs, skinless, boneless
- 1 teaspoon ground clove
- 1 tablespoon avocado oil
- ½ teaspoon ground black pepper
- 1 teaspoon cayenne pepper

Method:

1. In the shallow bowl, mix cayenne pepper, ground black pepper, and ground clove.

2. Rub the chicken thighs with the spice mixture and sprinkle with avocado oil.

3. Cook it in the slow cooker on saute mode for 10 minutes per side.

Nutritional info per serve: 286 calories, 42.4g protein, 0.9g carbohydrates, 11.5g fat, 0.5g fiber, 130mg cholesterol, 127mg sodium, 384mg potassium.

Garlic and Curry Chicken

Yield: 4 servings | **Prep time:** 10 minutes | **Cook time:** 5 hours

Ingredients:

- 1-pound chicken breast, skinless, boneless, chopped
- 1 teaspoon curry powder
- 1 cup coconut cream
- 1 teaspoon minced garlic
- 1 tablespoon coconut oil

Method:

1. Mix curry powder with coconut cream, and minced garlic.

2. Pour the liquid into the slow cooker bowl.

3. Add chicken breast and coconut oil.

4. Close the lid and cook the chicken on Low for 5 hours.

Nutritional info per serve: 299 calories, 25.5g protein, 3.8g carbohydrates, 20.6g fat, 1.5g fiber, 73mg cholesterol, 67mg sodium, 588mg potassium.

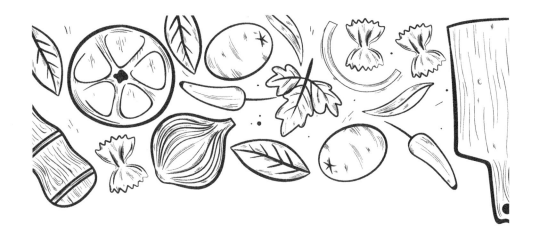

Fish and Seafood

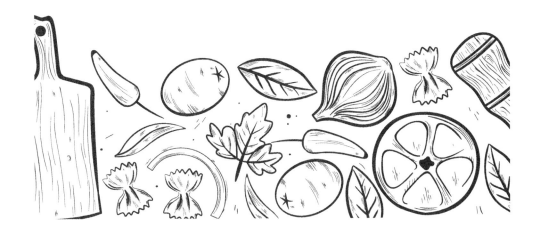

Tuna Pie

Yield: 6 servings | **Prep time:** 15 minutes | **Cook time:** 7 hours

Ingredients:
- 3 spring onions, chopped
- 1 cup coconut flour
- ¼ cup of coconut oil
- 1 egg, beaten
- 1 teaspoon baking powder
- 9 oz tuna, canned, shredded
- 1 cup of water, for cooking

Method:
1. In the mixing bowl mix baking powder with coconut oil, and coconut flour. Knead the dough and put it in the slow cooker baking mold. Flatten the dough in the shape of the pie crust.
2. Then mix shredded tuna with chopped spring onion and egg.
3. Put the fish mixture over the pie crust and flatten well.
4. Pour water into the slow cooker and insert the rack.
5. Put the pie on the rack and close the lid.
6. Cook the pie on low for 7 hours.

Nutritional info per serve: 181 calories, 12.7g protein, 2.3g carbohydrates, 13.6g fat, 1.1g fiber, 40mg cholesterol, 38mg sodium, 256mg potassium.

Wrapped Scallops

Yield: 4 servings | **Prep time:** 10 minutes | **Cook time:** 6 minutes

Ingredients:
- 1-pound scallops
- 5 oz bacon, sliced
- 1 teaspoon ground coriander
- ½ teaspoon avocado oil

Method:
1. Sprinkle the scallops with ground coriander and wrap in the bacon. Secure scallops with the help of the toothpicks if needed.
2. Preheat the avocado oil on saute mode for 2 minutes.
3. Then put the scallops in it.
4. Roast them for 3 minutes per side on saute mode.

Nutritional info per serve: 292 calories, 32.2g protein, 3.2g carbohydrates, 15.7g fat, 0g fiber, 76mg cholesterol, 1001mg sodium, 568mg potassium.

Lime Haddock

Yield: 4 servings | **Prep time:** 10 minutes | **Cook time:** 14 minutes

Ingredients:
- 1-pound haddock
- 1 tablespoon avocado oil
- 1 teaspoon ground black pepper
- 1 lime

Method:
1. Sprinkle the haddock with avocado oil, ground black pepper, and put in the slow cooker bowl.
2. Cut the lime into halves and squeeze over the fish.
3. Then sprinkle the fish with avocado oil and saute for 7 minutes per side on saute mode.

Nutritional info per serve: 138 calories, 27.7g protein, 2.3g carbohydrates, 1.5g fat, 0.8g fiber, 84mg cholesterol, 99mg sodium, 487mg potassium.

Cod in Sauce

Yield: 2 servings | **Prep time:** 10 minutes | **Cook time:** 3 hours

Ingredients:
- 1-pound cod fillet
- 1 teaspoon keto tomato paste
- ½ cup coconut cream
- 1 teaspoon curry paste

Method:
1. Mix coconut cream with curry paste, and keto tomato paste and pour in the slow cooker.
2. Add cod and cook the fish on High for 3 hours.

Nutritional info per serve: 340 calories, 42.1g protein, 4.6g carbohydrates, 17.8g fat, 1.5g fiber, 111mg cholesterol, 152mg sodium, 185mg potassium.

Soft Trout

Yield: 1 serving | **Prep time:** 10 minutes | **Cook time:** 14 minutes

Ingredients:
- 3 oz trout fillet
- 2 tablespoons coconut oil
- ¼ cup coconut cream
- 1 teaspoon ground black pepper

Method:
1. Sprinkle the trout fillet with coconut oil, coconut cream, and ground black pepper.
2. Put the fish in the slow cooker and cook it on saute mode for 7 minutes per side.

Nutritional info per serve: 539 calories, 24.3g protein, 4.7g carbohydrates, 48.8g fat, 1.9g fiber, 63mg cholesterol, 67mg sodium, 578mg potassium.

Lime Trout

Yield: 4 servings | **Prep time:** 15 minutes | **Cook time:** 1 hour

Ingredients:
- 4 trout fillets
- 1 lime
- 1 teaspoon dried thyme
- 1 teaspoon avocado oil
- 1 cup of water

Method:
1. Put the trout fillets and avocado oil in the slow cooker.
2. Add dried thyme and cook the fish on saute mode for 3 minutes per side.
3. Then add water.
4. Chop the lime and add it to the slow cooker too.
5. Close the lid and cook the trout on high for 1 hour.
6. Then top it with sliced lime and bake at 360F for 30 minutes.

Nutritional info per serve: 125 calories, 16.7g protein, 2g carbohydrates, 5.5g fat, 0.6g fiber, 46mg cholesterol, 44mg sodium, 310mg potassium.

Sour Cod

Yield: 4 servings | **Prep time:** 15 minutes | **Cook time:** 20 minutes

Ingredients:
- 1-pound cod, cut into medium-sized pieces
- ½ teaspoon chives, chopped
- 2 tablespoons coconut aminos
- 1 teaspoon dried dill
- ½ teaspoon lemon zest, grated
- 1 teaspoon avocado oil

Method:
1. Put the cod in the big bowl and sprinkle it with chives, coconut aminos, dried dill, and lemon zest.
2. Add avocado oil and carefully mix the fish. Leave it for 10 minutes to marinate.
3. Preheat the slow cooker bowl for 4 minutes on saute mode.
4. Add the cod and cook it on saute mode for 6 minutes per side.

Nutritional info per serve: 129 calories, 26g protein, 1.8g carbohydrates, 1.1g fat, 0.1g fiber, 62mg cholesterol, 98mg sodium, 290mg potassium.

Parmesan Cod

Yield: 4 servings | **Prep time:** 10 minutes | **Cook time:** 16 minutes

Ingredients:
- 2 oz Parmesan cheese, grated
- 1 teaspoon olive oil
- ½ teaspoon cayenne pepper
- 4 cod fillets

Method:
1. Brush the cod fillets with olive oil from each side and sprinkle with cayenne pepper.
2. Put the fish in the slow cooker bowl and cook on saute mode for 8 minutes per side.

Nutritional info per serve: 146 calories, 24.6g protein, 0.6g carbohydrates, 5.3g fat, 0.1g fiber, 65mg cholesterol, 202mg sodium, 5mg potassium.

Cod with Chives

Yield: 4 servings | **Prep time:** 10 minutes | **Cook time:** 3 hours

Ingredients:
- 4 cod fillets
- ½ lemon
- 1 rosemary, fresh
- 1 oz chives, chopped
- ½ cup coconut cream

Method:
1. Put all ingredients in the slow cooker and close the lid.
2. Cook the fish on High for 3 hours.

Nutritional info per serve: 164 calories, 21g protein, 2.8g carbohydrates, 8.3g fat, 1.2g fiber, 55mg cholesterol, 75mg sodium, 113mg potassium.

Italian Spices Seabass

Yield: 4 servings | **Prep time:** 10 minutes | **Cook time:** 5 hours

Ingredients:
- 1-pound seabass
- 2 tablespoons butter, softened
- 1 tablespoon Italian seasonings

Method:
1. Rub the seabass with butter and Italian seasonings. Wrap it in the foil and put it in the slow cooker.
2. Cook it on low for 5 hours.

Nutritional info per serve: 119 calories, 0.1g protein, 1.9g carbohydrates, 8.3g fat, 0g fiber, 18mg cholesterol, 155mg sodium, 3mg potassium.

Cheddar Tilapia

Yield: 4 servings | **Prep time:** 10 minutes | **Cook time:** 20 minutes

Ingredients:

- 4 tilapia fillets, boneless
- ½ cup Cheddar cheese, shredded
- 1 teaspoon lemon juice
- 1 teaspoon dried thyme
- 1 teaspoon avocado oil

Method:

1. Rub the tilapia fillets with dried thyme. Sprinkle it with avocado oil.
2. Put them in the slow cooker bowl.
3. After this, sprinkle the fish with lemon juice and shredded cheese.
4. Close the lid and saute the fish for 20 minutes on saute mode.

Nutritional info per serve: 152 calories, 24.6g protein, 0.4g carbohydrates, 5.9g fat, 0.2g fiber, 70mg cholesterol, 128mg sodium, 21mg potassium.

Cinnamon Hake

Yield: 4 servings | **Prep time:** 10 minutes | **Cook time:** 10 minutes

Ingredients:

- 4 hake fillets
- ½ teaspoon ground cinnamon
- 1 tablespoon coconut oil, melted
- ½ teaspoon chili powder

Method:

1. Brush the slow cooker mold with coconut oil and put the hake fillets inside one layer.
2. Sprinkle the fish with ground cinnamon and chili powder.
3. Cook it on saute mode for 5 minutes per side.

Nutritional info per serve: 145 calories, 25.5g protein, 1.7g carbohydrates, 4.7g fat, 0.3g fiber, 51mg cholesterol, 232mg sodium, 8mg potassium.

Salmon Kababs

Yield: 4 servings | **Prep time:** 15 minutes | **Cook time:** 2 hours

Ingredients:

- 1-pound salmon fillet
- 1 tablespoon marinara sauce
- 1 teaspoon avocado oil
- ¼ teaspoon ground cumin
- 1 cup of water, for cooking

Method:

1. Cut the salmon fillet into medium cubes and mix with marinara sauce, avocado oil, and ground cumin.
2. String the fish cubes in the skewers.
3. Insert the rack in the slow cooker and add water.
4. Put the salmon skewers on the rack and close the lid.
5. Cook the kababs on high for 2 hours.

Nutritional info per serve: 155 calories, 22.1g protein, 0.7g carbohydrates, 7.3g fat, 0.2g fiber, 50mg cholesterol, 66mg sodium, 454mg potassium.

Spicy Salmon

Yield: 4 servings | **Prep time:** 10 minutes | **Cook time:** 20 minutes

Ingredients:

- 2 tablespoons coconut oil, softened
- 1¼ pound salmon fillet
- 1 teaspoon chili powder

Method:

1. Sprinkle the salmon fillet with chili powder.
2. Then melt the coconut oil in the slow cooker on saute mode.
3. Add salmon and saute it for 6 minutes per side.

Nutritional info per serve: 473 calories, 60.6g protein, 0.4g carbohydrates, 26.2g fat, 0.2g fiber, 138mg cholesterol, 144mg sodium, 1210mg potassium.

Oregano Salmon

Yield: 3 servings | **Prep time:** 10 minutes | **Cook time:** 10 minutes

Ingredients:

- 3 salmon fillets
- 1 teaspoon dried oregano
- 1 tablespoon avocado oil

Method:

1. Rub the salmon fillets with dried oregano.
2. Then preheat the slow cooker for 3 minutes on saute mode.
3. Add avocado oil and salmon.
4. Saute it for 4 minutes per side on saute mode.

Nutritional info per serve: 243 calories, 34.7g protein, 0.6g carbohydrates, 11.6g fat, 0.4g fiber, 78mg cholesterol, 79mg sodium, 707mg potassium.

Tilapia Bowl

Yield: 4 servings | **Prep time:** 10 minutes | **Cook time:** 10 minutes

Ingredients:

- 9 oz tilapia fillet, chopped
- ½ cup white cabbage, shredded
- 1 teaspoon coconut oil
- 1 teaspoon chili powder
- ½ teaspoon cayenne pepper
- 1 cup coconut cream

Method:

1. Melt the coconut oil in on the saute mode.
2. Add tilapia and chili powder. Roast the fish for 2 minutes on saute mode.
3. Then add cayenne pepper and cook the fish for 1 minute more.
4. Transfer the cooked tilapia into the bowl.
5. Add shredded cabbage and coconut cream.
6. Carefully mix the meal.

Nutritional info per serve: 205 calories, 13.5g protein, 4.3g carbohydrates, 16.2g fat, 1.8g fiber, 31mg cholesterol, 40mg sodium, 190mg potassium.

Cod Curry

Yield: 6 servings | **Prep time:** 10 minutes | **Cook time:** 6 hours

Ingredients:

- 1-pound cod fillet, chopped
- 1 tablespoon curry paste
- ½ teaspoon dried cilantro
- 1 teaspoon chili
- powder
- ½ bell pepper, diced
- 1 teaspoon coconut oil
- ½ cup coconut cream
- ½ teaspoon keto tomato paste

Method:

1. In the mixing bowl, mix keto tomato paste with coconut cream, chili powder, dried cilantro, and curry paste.
2. Then add cod and carefully mix the mixture. Add bell pepper and mix the mixture again.
3. Transfer the mixture to the slow cooker and close the lid.
4. Cook the cod on low for 6 hours.

Nutritional info per serve: 135 calories, 14.3g protein, 2.9g carbohydrates, 7.8g fat, 0.7g fiber, 37mg cholesterol, 55mg sodium, 84mg potassium.

Salmon Meatballs

Yield: 4 servings | **Prep time:** 10 minutes | **Cook time:** 10 minutes

Ingredients:

- 10 oz salmon, minced
- 1 teaspoon minced garlic
- 2 tablespoons coconut flour
- ½ teaspoon dried oregano
- ½ teaspoon dried cilantro
- 1 tablespoon coconut oil

Method:

1. In the mixing bowl, mix minced salmon, minced garlic, coconut flour, dried oregano, and cilantro.
2. Make the fish balls from the mixture.
3. Then preheat the coconut oil on saute mode.
4. Add fish meatballs and roast them for 4 minutes per side on saute mode or until they are light brown.

Nutritional info per serve: 155 calories, 14.8g protein, 4.4g carbohydrates, 8.1g fat, 2.6g fiber, 31mg cholesterol, 46mg sodium, 278mg potassium.

Parsley Tuna Fritters

Yield: 8 servings | **Prep time:** 10 minutes | **Cook time:** 20 minutes

Ingredients:

- 12 ounces canned tuna, drained well and flaked
- 2 tablespoons fresh parsley, chopped
- 1 egg, beaten
- 2 tablespoons coconut oil
- 2 tablespoons coconut flour
- ½ teaspoon ground cumin

Method:

1. In the mixing bowl, mix canned tuna with parsley, egg, coconut flour, and cumin.
2. Then make the small fritters from the tuna mixture.
3. Melt the coconut oil in the slow cooker on saute mode.
4. Add the tuna fritters and roast them for 4 minutes per side on saute mode.

Nutritional info per serve: 132 calories, 12.5g protein, 2.2g carbohydrates, 7.9g fat, 1.3g fiber, 34mg cholesterol, 37mg sodium, 157mg potassium.

Sage Cod Fillets

Yield: 2 servings | **Prep time:** 10 minutes | **Cook time:** 15 minutes

Ingredients:

- 2 cod fillets
- 1 teaspoon dried sage
- 1 tablespoon coconut
- aminos
- 1 tablespoon avocado oil

Method:

1. Mix dried sage with coconut aminos and avocado oil.

2. Then mix fish with coconut aminos mixture and leave for 10 minutes to marinate.

3. Put the cod fillets in the slow cooker and close the lid.

4. Saute them for 15 minutes on saute mode.

Nutritional info per serve: 108 calories, 20.1g protein, 2.1g carbohydrates, 1.9g fat, 0.4g fiber, 55mg cholesterol, 79mg sodium, 26mg potassium.

Salmon Boats

Yield: 6 servings | **Prep time:** 10 minutes | **Cook time:** 7 minutes

Ingredients:

- 6 celery stalks
- 8 oz salmon fillet
- 1 teaspoon olive oil
- 1 teaspoon scallions, chopped
- 1 tablespoon ricotta cheese

Method:

1. Preheat the olive oil on saute mode for 3 minutes.

2. Then add salmon fillet and roast it for 2 minutes per side.

3. After this, shred the salmon and mix it with scallions and ricotta cheese.

4. Then fill the celery with a salmon mixture.

Nutritional info per serve: 63 calories, 7.8g protein, 0.7g carbohydrates, 3.3g fat, 0.3g fiber, 17mg cholesterol, 34mg sodium, 193mg potassium.

Herbed Oysters

Yield: 6 servings | **Prep time:** 10 minutes | **Cook time:** 10 minutes

Ingredients:

- 6 oysters, shucked
- 1 teaspoon Italian seasonings
- 1 tablespoon dried cilantro
- 1 tablespoon coconut oil

Method:

1. Melt the coconut oil on saute mode and add oysters.

2. Sprinkle them with Italian seasonings and dried cilantro and roast for 7 minutes on saute mode.

Nutritional info per serve: 122 calories, 10g protein, 6.1g carbohydrates, 6.5g fat, 0g fiber, 81mg cholesterol, 300mg sodium, 1mg potassium.

Roasted Sea Eel

Yield: 4 servings | **Prep time:** 10 minutes | **Cook time:** 15 minutes

Ingredients:

- 10 oz sea eel
- 1 teaspoon cayenne pepper
- ½ teaspoon ground paprika
- ½ teaspoon chili flakes
- ½ teaspoon keto tomato paste
- 2 oz celery stalk, chopped
- 1 teaspoon coconut oil

Method:

1. Melt the coconut oil on saute mode.

2. Add sea eel and sprinkle it with cayenne pepper, ground paprika, chili flakes, and celery stalk.

3. Add keto tomato paste and carefully mix the mixture.

4. Cook it for 10 minutes on saute mode.

5. Then flip it on another side and cook for 5 minutes more.

Nutritional info per serve: 157 calories, 6.5g protein, 9.8g carbohydrates, 6g fat, 0.5g fiber, 49mg cholesterol, 259mg sodium, 60mg potassium.

Shrimp Chowder

Yield: 5 servings | **Prep time:** 10 minutes | **Cook time:** 1 hour

Ingredients:

- 7 oz cod fillet, chopped
- 5 oz shrimps, peeled
- 1 oz pancetta, chopped
- 1 spring onion, diced
- ½ cup celery stalk
- ½ cup heavy cream
- 3 cups of water

Method:

1. Roast the pancetta on saute mode for 2 minutes per side.

2. Then add all remaining ingredients and carefully mix.

3. Cook the chowder on saute mode for 1 hour.

Nutritional info per serve: 140 calories, 16g protein, 1.4g carbohydrates, 7.7g fat, 0.2g fiber, 102mg cholesterol, 242mg sodium, 125mg potassium.

Cilantro Salmon

Yield: 4 servings | **Prep time:** 10 minutes | **Cook time:** 10 minutes

Prep time: 10 minutes

Cook time: 8 minutes

Servings: 4

Ingredients:

- ½ teaspoon garlic powder
- 1-pound salmon fillet
- 1 tablespoon avocado oil
- 1 tablespoon dried cilantro

Method:

1. Sprinkle the salmon fillet with avocado oil, dried cilantro, and garlic powder.
2. Cook the fish on saute mode for 5 minutes per side.

Nutritional info per serve: 156 calories, 22.1g protein, 0.5g carbohydrates, 7.4g fat, 0.2g fiber, 50mg cholesterol, 50mg sodium, 452mg potassium.

Mustard Cod

Yield: 4 servings | **Prep time:** 10 minutes | **Cook time:** 3 hours

Ingredients:

- 4 cod fillets
- 1 tablespoon mustard
- 1 cup coconut milk
- 1 teaspoon avocado oil

Method:

1. Mix mustard with coconut milk.
2. Then mix cod fillets with mustard mixture and leave for 10 minutes to marinate.
3. Pour avocado oil into the slow cooker.
4. Add fish mixture and close the lid.
5. Cook the meal for 3 hours on High.

Nutritional info per serve: 243 calories, 22.1g protein, 4.4g carbohydrates, 16.3g fat, 1.8g fiber, 55mg cholesterol, 79mg sodium, 181mg potassium.

Onion Salmon

Yield: 4 servings | **Prep time:** 10 minutes | **Cook time:** 4 hours

Ingredients:

- 4 salmon fillets
- 1 tablespoon avocado oil
- 1 teaspoon ground coriander
- 1 teaspoon sweet paprika
- 2 scallions, diced
- 1 teaspoon onion powder

Method:

1. In the mixing bowl, mix salmon fillets with avocado oil, ground coriander, sweet paprika, and onion powder.
2. Put the mixture in the slow cooker bowl.
3. Then top the fish with scallions and cover with foil.
4. Close the lid and cook the salmon on Low for 4 hours.

Nutritional info per serve: 246 calories, 34.9g protein, 1.5g carbohydrates, 11.5g fat, 0.6g fiber, 78mg cholesterol, 80mg sodium, 734mg potassium.

Cheddar Pollock

Yield: 3 servings | **Prep time:** 10 minutes | **Cook time:** 2 hours

Ingredients:

- 11 oz Pollock fillet
- ½ cup Cheddar cheese, shredded
- 1 teaspoon white
- pepper
- 1 tablespoon avocado oil
- 1 cup heavy cream

Method:

1. Put all ingredients in the slow cooker.
2. Close the lid and cook the fish on high for 2 hours.

Nutritional info per serve: 315 calories, 26.1g protein, 2.1g carbohydrates, 22.6g fat, 0.4g fiber, 126mg cholesterol, 193mg sodium, 72mg potassium.

Sweet Milkfish Saute

Yield: 4 servings | **Prep time:** 10 minutes | **Cook time:** 3 hours

Ingredients:

- 1 tablespoon Erythritol
- 12 oz milkfish fillet, chopped
- 2 tomatoes, chopped
- ½ cup of water
- 1 teaspoon ground cardamom

Method:

1. Mix Erythritol with tomatoes and ground cardamom.
2. Transfer the ingredients to the slow cooker.
3. Then add milkfish fillet and water.
4. Cook the saute on High for 3 hours.
5. Carefully stir the saute before serving.

Nutritional info per serve: 174 calories, 23g protein, 6.5g carbohydrates, 7.5g fat, 0.9g fiber, 57mg cholesterol, 82mg sodium, 470mg potassium.

Clam Stew

Yield: 3 servings | **Prep time:** 5 minutes | **Cook time:** 30 minutes

Ingredients:
- 5 oz clams
- ½ cup heavy cream
- ½ teaspoon curry paste
- ½ cup bell pepper, chopped
- 1 teaspoon keto tomato paste
- 1 cup of water
- 8 oz shrimps, peeled

Method:
1. Put all ingredients in the slow cooker and cook on High for 30 minutes.

Nutritional info per serve: 195 calories, 18.2g protein, 9g carbohydrates, 9.3g fat, 0.6g fiber, 187mg cholesterol, 367mg sodium, 242mg potassium.

Fish Pie

Yield: 6 servings | **Prep time:** 15 minutes | **Cook time:** 7 hours

Ingredients:
- 7 oz keto dough
- 1 tablespoon cream cheese
- 8 oz salmon fillet, chopped
- 1 yellow onion, diced
- 1 tablespoon fresh dill
- 1 teaspoon olive oil

Method:
1. Brush the slow cooker bottom with olive oil.
2. Then roll up the dough and place it in the slow cooker.
3. Flatten it in the shape of the pie crust.
4. After this, in the mixing bowl mix cream cheese, salmon, onion, and dill.
5. Put the fish mixture over the pie crust and cover it with foil.
6. Close the lid and cook the pie on Low for 7 hours.

Nutritional info per serve: 189 calories, 26.9g protein, 9.4g carbohydrates, 5.2g fat, 4.9g fiber, 19mg cholesterol, 163mg sodium, 191mg potassium.

Fennel Seabass

Yield: 4 servings | **Prep time:** 10 minutes | **Cook time:** 5 hours

Ingredients:
- 1-pound seabass
- 1 tablespoon fennel seeds
- 1 teaspoon avocado oil
- 1 teaspoon minced garlic

Method:
1. In the shallow bowl, mix fennel seeds with avocado oil, and minced garlic.
2. Then carefully rub the seabass with fennel mixture and wrap it in the foil.
3. Put the fish in the slow cooker and cook it on Low for 5 hours.

Nutritional info per serve: 65 calories, 0.3g protein, 2.6g carbohydrates, 1.9g fat, 0.6g fiber, 0mg cholesterol, 114mg sodium, 31mg potassium.

Onion Cod Fillets

Yield: 4 servings | **Prep time:** 10 minutes | **Cook time:** 3 hours

Ingredients:
- 1 onion, minced
- 4 cod fillets
- 1 teaspoon dried cilantro
- ½ cup of water
- 1 teaspoon coconut oil, melted

Method:
1. Sprinkle the cod fillets with dried cilantro, and coconut oil.
2. Then place them in the slow cooker and top with minced onion.
3. Add water and close the lid.
4. Cook the fish on high for 3 hours.

Nutritional info per serve: 109 calories, 20.3g protein, 2.6g carbohydrates, 2g fat, 0.6g fiber, 58mg cholesterol, 660mg sodium, 41mg potassium

Tender Tilapia in Cream Sauce

Yield: 4 servings | **Prep time:** 10 minutes | **Cook time:** 5 hours

Ingredients:
- 4 tilapia fillets
- ½ cup heavy cream
- 1 teaspoon garlic powder
- 1 teaspoon ground black pepper
- 1 teaspoon almond flour

Method:
1. Mix almond flour with cream until smooth.
2. Then pour the liquid into the slow cooker.
3. After this, sprinkle the tilapia fillets with garlic powder, and ground black pepper.
4. Place the fish fillets in the slow cooker and close the lid.
5. Cook the fish on Low for 5 hours.

Nutritional info per serve: 151 calories, 21.6g protein, 1.7g carbohydrates, 6.6g fat, 0.3g fiber, 76mg cholesterol, 337mg sodium, 28mg potassium

Lemon Scallops

Yield: 4 servings | **Prep time:** 10 minutes | **Cook time:** 1 hour

Ingredients:
- 1-pound scallops
- 1 teaspoon ground white pepper
- ½ teaspoon olive oil
- 3 tablespoons lemon juice
- 1 teaspoon lemon zest, grated
- 1 tablespoon dried oregano
- ½ cup of water

Method:
1. Sprinkle the scallops with ground white pepper, lemon juice, and lemon zest and leave for 10-15 minutes to marinate.
2. After this, sprinkle the scallops with olive oil and dried oregano.
3. Put the scallops in the slow cooker and add water.
4. Cook the seafood on High for 1 hour.

Nutritional info per serve: 113 calories, 19.3g protein, 4.1g carbohydrates, 1.7g fat, 0.7g fiber, 37mg cholesterol, 768mg sodium, 407mg potassium

Haddock Chowder

Yield: 5 servings | **Prep time:** 10 minutes | **Cook time:** 6 hours

Ingredients:
- 1-pound haddock, chopped
- 2 bacon slices, chopped, cooked
- ½ cup cauliflower, chopped
- 1 teaspoon ground coriander
- ½ cup heavy cream
- 4 cups of water

Method:
1. Put all ingredients in the slow cooker and close the lid.
2. Cook the chowder on Low for 6 hours.

Nutritional info per serve: 203 calories, 27.1g protein, 2.8g carbohydrates, 8.6g fat, 0.4g fiber, 97mg cholesterol, 737mg sodium, 506mg potassium

Shrimp Scampi

Yield: 4 servings | **Prep time:** 5 minutes | **Cook time:** 4 hours

Ingredients:
- 1-pound shrimps, peeled
- 2 tablespoons lemon juice
- 2 tablespoons coconut oil
- 1 cup of water
- 1 teaspoon dried parsley
- ½ teaspoon white pepper

Method:
1. Put all ingredients in the slow cooker and gently mix.
2. Close the lid and cook the scampi on Low for 4 hours.

Nutritional info per serve: 196 calories, 25.9g protein, 2.1g carbohydrates, 8.8g fat, 0.1g fiber, 239mg cholesterol, 280mg sodium, 207mg potassium

Nutmeg Trout

Yield: 4 servings | **Prep time:** 10 minutes | **Cook time:** 3 hours

Ingredients:
- 1 tablespoon ground nutmeg
- 1 tablespoon coconut oil, softened
- 1 teaspoon dried cilantro
- 1 teaspoon dried oregano
- 1 teaspoon keto fish sauce
- 4 trout fillets
- ½ cup of water

Method:
1. In the shallow bowl mix coconut oil with cilantro, dried oregano, and fish sauce. Add ground nutmeg and whisk the mixture.
2. Then grease the fish fillets with a nutmeg mixture and put them in the slow cooker.
3. Add remaining coconut oil mixture and water.
4. Cook the fish on high for 3 hours.

Nutritional info per serve: 154 calories, 16.8g protein, 1.2g carbohydrates, 8.8g fat, 0.5g fiber, 54mg cholesterol, 178mg sodium, 305mg potassium.

Clams in Coconut Sauce

Yield: 4 servings | **Prep time:** 10 minutes | **Cook time:** 2 hours

Ingredients:
- 1 cup coconut cream
- 1 teaspoon minced garlic
- 1 teaspoon chili flakes
- 1 teaspoon ground coriander
- 8 oz clams

Method:
1. Pour coconut cream into the slow cooker.
2. Add minced garlic, chili flakes, and ground coriander.
3. Cook the mixture on high for 1 hour.
4. Then add clams and stir the meal well. Cook it for 1 hour on high more.

Nutritional info per serve: 166 calories, 1.8g protein, 9.8g carbohydrates, 14.4g fat, 1.6g fiber, 0mg cholesterol, 214mg sodium, 212mg potassium

Thyme Mussels

Yield: 4 servings | **Prep time:** 10 minutes | **Cook time:** 2.5 hours

Ingredients:
- 1-pound mussels
- 1 teaspoon dried thyme
- 1 teaspoon ground

- black pepper
- 1 cup of water
- ½ cup Greek yogurt

Method:
1. In the mixing bowl mix mussels, dried thyme, and ground black pepper.
2. Then pour water into the slow cooker.
3. Add Greek yogurt and cook the liquid on High for 1.5 hours.
4. After this, add mussels and cook them for 1 hour on High or until the mussels are opened.

Nutritional info per serve: 161 calories, 14.5g protein, 5.9g carbohydrates, 8.6g fat, 0.2g fiber, 44mg cholesterol, 632mg sodium, 414mg potassium.

Cinnamon Catfish

Yield: 2 servings | **Prep time:** 10 minutes | **Cook time:** 2.5 hours

Ingredients:
- 2 catfish fillets
- 1 teaspoon ground cinnamon
- 1 tablespoon lemon

- juice
- ½ teaspoon avocado oil
- 1/3 cup water

Method:
1. Sprinkle the fish fillets with ground cinnamon, lemon juice, and avocado oil.
2. Put the fillets in the slow cooker in one layer.
3. Add water and close the lid.
4. Cook the meal on High for 2.5 hours.

Nutritional info per serve: 231 calories, 25g protein, 1.1g carbohydrates, 13.3g fat, 0.6g fiber, 75mg cholesterol, 88mg sodium, 528mg potassium.

Hot Salmon

Yield: 4 servings | **Prep time:** 10 minutes | **Cook time:** 3 hours

Ingredients:
- 1-pound salmon fillet, sliced
- 2 chili peppers, chopped

- 1 tablespoon olive oil
- 1 onion, diced
- ½ cup coconut cream

Method:
1. Mix salmon with onion and olive oil.
2. Transfer the ingredients to the slow cooker.
3. Add coconut cream and onion.
4. Cook the salmon on high for 3 hours.

Nutritional info per serve: 211 calories, 22.6g protein, 3.7g carbohydrates, 12.2g fat, 0.7g fiber, 56mg cholesterol, 352mg sodium, 491mg potassium.

Sage Shrimps

Yield: 4 servings | **Prep time:** 10 minutes | **Cook time:** 1 hour

Ingredients:
- 1-pound shrimps, peeled
- 1 teaspoon dried sage
- 1 teaspoon minced garlic

- 1 teaspoon white pepper
- 2 tomatoes chopped
- ½ cup of water

Method:
1. Put all ingredients in the slow cooker and close the lid.
2. Cook the shrimps on High for 1 hour.

Nutritional info per serve: 146 calories, 26.4g protein, 4.1g carbohydrates, 2.1g fat, 0.8g fiber, 239mg cholesterol, 280mg sodium, 310mg potassium.

Cumin Snapper

Yield: 4 servings | **Prep time:** 15 minutes | **Cook time:** 4 hours

Ingredients:
- 1-pound snapper, peeled, cleaned
- 1 teaspoon ground cumin
- ½ teaspoon garlic powder

- 1 teaspoon dried oregano
- 1 tablespoon avocado oil
- ¼ cup of water

Method:
1. Cut the snapper into 4 servings.
2. After this, in the shallow bowl mix ground cumin, garlic powder, and dried oregano.
3. Sprinkle fish with spices and avocado oil.
4. Arrange the snapper in the slow cooker. Add water.
5. Cook the fish on Low for 4 hours.

Nutritional info per serve: 183 calories, 29.9g protein, 0.7g carbohydrates, 5.6g fat, 0.3g fiber, 54mg cholesterol, 360mg sodium, 20mg potassium.

Fish Salpicao

Yield: 4 servings | **Prep time:** 5 minutes | **Cook time:** 1 hour

Ingredients:

- 1 teaspoon ground black pepper
- 1 teaspoon cayenne pepper
- 1 tablespoon avocado oil
- 1-pound cod fillet
- 1 garlic clove, diced

Method:

1. Put all ingredients in the slow cooker and carefully mix.
2. Then close the lid and cook the meal on High for 1 hour.

Nutritional info per serve: 100 calories, 20.5g protein, 1g carbohydrates, 1.6g fat, 0.4g fiber, 56mg cholesterol, 653mg sodium, 30mg potassium.

Miso Cod

Yield: 4 servings | **Prep time:** 10 minutes | **Cook time:** 4 hours

Ingredients:

- 1-pound cod fillet, sliced
- 1 teaspoon keto miso paste
- ½ teaspoon ground
- ginger
- 2 cups chicken stock
- ½ teaspoon ground nutmeg

Method:

1. In the mixing bowl mix chicken stock, ground nutmeg, ground ginger, and miso paste.
2. Then pour the liquid into the slow cooker.
3. Add cod fillet and close the lid.
4. Cook the fish on Low for 4 hours.

Nutritional info per serve: 101 calories, 20.8g protein, 1.1g carbohydrates, 1.5g fat, 0.2g fiber, 56mg cholesterol, 506mg sodium, 14mg potassium.

Coconut Catfish

Yield: 3 servings | **Prep time:** 10 minutes | **Cook time:** 2.5 hours

Ingredients:

- 3 catfish fillets
- 1 teaspoon coconut shred
- ½ cup of coconut milk
- 12 tablespoons keto fish sauce
- 1 cup of water
- 2 tablespoons keto soy sauce

Method:

1. Pour water into the slow cooker.
2. Add soy sauce, fish sauce, and coconut milk.
3. Then add coconut shred and catfish fillets.
4. Cook the fish on high for 2.5 hours.

Nutritional info per serve: 329 calories, 27.3g protein, 3.9g carbohydrates, 22.7g fat, 1.2g fiber, 75mg cholesterol, 1621mg sodium, 682mg potassium.

Hot Calamari

Yield: 4 servings | **Prep time:** 10 minutes | **Cook time:** 1 hour

Ingredients:

- 12 oz calamari, sliced
- ¼ cup of soy sauce
- 1 teaspoon cayenne pepper
- 1 garlic clove,
- crushed
- 1 teaspoon mustard
- ½ cup of water
- 1 teaspoon avocado oil

Method:

1. In the bowl mix slices of calamari, soy sauce, cayenne pepper, garlic, mustard, and avocado oil. Leave the ingredients for 10 minutes to marinate.
2. Then transfer the mixture to the slow cooker, add water, and close the lid.
3. Cook the meal on high for 1 hour.

Nutritional info per serve: 103 calories, 14.6g protein, 4.6g carbohydrates, 2.6g fat, 0.4g fiber, 198mg cholesterol, 937mg sodium, 262mg potassium.

Curry Squid

Yield: 5 servings | **Prep time:** 10 minutes | **Cook time:** 3 hours

Ingredients:

- 15 oz squid, peeled, sliced
- 1 teaspoon curry paste
- ½ cup of coconut
- milk
- ¼ cup of water
- 1 teaspoon dried dill
- 1 teaspoon ground nutmeg

Method:

1. Mix coconut milk with water and curry paste.
2. Then pour the liquid into the slow cooker.
3. Add dried dill and ground nutmeg.
4. After this, add the sliced squid and close the lid.
5. Cook the meal on low for 3 hours.

Nutritional info per serve: 143 calories, 13.9g protein, 4.6g carbohydrates, 7.6g fat, 0.7g fiber, 198mg cholesterol, 42mg sodium, 281mg potassium.

Rosemary Seabass

Yield: 3 servings | **Prep time:** 10 minutes | **Cook time:** 4 hours

Ingredients:

- 3 seabass fillets
- 1 teaspoon dried rosemary
- 2 teaspoons avocado oil
- ½ cup of water

Method:

1. Rub the seabass fillets with dried rosemary and avocado oil.
2. Then place them in the slow cooker in one layer.
3. Add water and close the lid.
4. Cook the fish on low for 4 hours.

Nutritional info per serve: 271 calories, 26.3g protein, 2.3g carbohydrates, 17.2g fat, 1.6g fiber, 0mg cholesterol, 16mg sodium, 69mg potassium.

Butter Salmon

Yield: 2 servings | **Prep time:** 10 minutes | **Cook time:** 1.5 hours

Ingredients:

- 8 oz salmon fillet
- 3 tablespoons butter
- 1 teaspoon dried sage
- ¼ cup of water

Method:

1. Churn butter with sage and preheat the mixture until liquid.
2. Then cut the salmon fillets into 2 servings and put them in the slow cooker.
3. Add water and melted butter mixture.
4. Close the lid and cook the salmon on High for 1.5 hours.

Nutritional info per serve: 304 calories, 22.2g protein, 0.2g carbohydrates, 24.3g fat, 0.1g fiber, 96mg cholesterol, 174mg sodium, 444mg potassium.

Cod Sticks

Yield: 2 servings | **Prep time:** 15 minutes | **Cook time:** 1.5 hour

Ingredients:

- 2 cod fillets
- 1 teaspoon ground black pepper
- 1 egg, beaten
- 1/3 cup coconut shred
- 1 tablespoon coconut oil
- ¼ cup of water

Method:

1. Cut the cod fillets into medium sticks and sprinkle with ground black pepper.
2. Then dip the fish in the beaten egg and coat it in the coconut shred.
3. Pour water into the slow cooker.
4. Add coconut oil and fish sticks.
5. Cook the meal on High for 1.5 hours.

Nutritional info per serve: 272 calories, 23.8g protein, 4.4g carbohydrates, 18.9g fat, 2.1g fiber, 137mg cholesterol, 107mg sodium, 43mg potassium.

Cardamom Trout

Yield: 4 servings | **Prep time:** 10 minutes | **Cook time:** 2.5 hours

Ingredients:

- 1 teaspoon ground cardamom
- 1-pound trout fillet
- 1 teaspoon butter, melted
- 1 tablespoon lemon juice
- ¼ cup of water

Method:

1. In the shallow bowl mix butter, and lemon juice.
2. Then sprinkle the trout fillet with ground cardamom and butter mixture.
3. Place the fish in the slow cooker and add water.
4. Cook the meal on High for 2.5 hours.

Nutritional info per serve: 226 calories, 30.3g protein, 0.4g carbohydrates, 10.6g fat, 0.2g fiber, 86mg cholesterol, 782mg sodium, 536mg potassium.

Rosemary Sole

Yield: 2 servings | **Prep time:** 10 minutes | **Cook time:** 2 hours

Ingredients:

- 8 oz sole fillet
- 1 tablespoon dried rosemary
- 1 tablespoon avocado oil
- 1 tablespoon apple cider vinegar
- 5 tablespoons water

Method:

1. Pour water into the slow cooker.
2. Then rub the sole fillet with dried rosemary and sprinkle with avocado oil and apple cider vinegar.
3. Put the fish fillet in the slow cooker and cook it on High for 2 hours.

Nutritional info per serve: 149 calories, 27.6g protein, 1.5g carbohydrates, 2.9g fat, 1g fiber, 77mg cholesterol, 122mg sodium, 434mg potassium.

Cheesy Fish Dip

Yield: 6 servings | **Prep time:** 10 minutes | **Cook time:** 5 hours

Ingredients:

- ½ cup coconut cream
- ½ cup Mozzarella, shredded
- 8 oz tuna, canned, shredded
- 2 oz chives, chopped

Method:

1. Put all ingredients in the slow cooker and gently mix.
2. Then close the lid and cook the fish dip in Low for 5 hours.

Nutritional info per serve: 93 calories, 11.2g protein, 1.1g carbohydrates, 4.7g fat, 0.2g fiber, 17mg cholesterol, 40mg sodium, 161mg potassium.

Seabass Balls

Yield: 4 servings | **Prep time:** 20 minutes | **Cook time:** 2 hours

Ingredients:

- 1 teaspoon ground coriander
- 2 tablespoons coconut flour
- ½ cup chicken stock
- 1 teaspoon dried dill
- 10 oz seabass fillet
- 1 tablespoon avocado oil

Method:

1. Dice the seabass fillet into tiny pieces and mix with ground coriander, coconut flour, and dill.
2. Make the medium size balls.
3. Preheat the skillet well.
4. Add avocado oil and heat it until hot.
5. Add the fish balls and roast them on high heat for 1 minute per side.
6. Then transfer the fish balls to the slow cooker. Arrange them in one layer.
7. Add water and close the lid.
8. Cook the meal on High for 2 hours.

Nutritional info per serve: 191 calories, 16.6g protein, 3.2g carbohydrates, 12.2g fat, 0.7g fiber, 0mg cholesterol, 387mg sodium, 15mg potassium.

Tuna Casserole

Yield: 4 servings | **Prep time:** 15 minutes | **Cook time:** 7 hours

Ingredients:

- 1 cup mushrooms, sliced
- 8 oz tuna, chopped
- 1 teaspoon Italian seasonings
- 1 cup chicken stock
- ½ cup Cheddar cheese, shredded
- 1 tablespoon avocado oil

Method:

1. Heat the avocado oil in the skillet.
2. Add mushrooms and roast them for 5 minutes on medium heat.
3. Then transfer the mushrooms to the slow cooker and flatten in one layer.
4. After this, mix Italian seasonings with tuna and put them over the mushrooms.
5. Then top the fish with cheese.
6. Add chicken stock.
7. Cook the casserole on Low for 7 hours.

Nutritional info per serve: 219 calories, 19.9g protein, 4.7g carbohydrates, 13.4g fat, 0.7g fiber, 33mg cholesterol, 311mg sodium, 315mg potassium.

Lemon Trout

Yield: 4 servings | **Prep time:** 15 minutes | **Cook time:** 5 hours

Ingredients:

- 1-pound trout, peeled, cleaned
- 1 lemon, sliced
- 1 teaspoon dried thyme
- 1 teaspoon ground black pepper
- 1 tablespoon olive oil
- ½ cup of water

Method:

1. Rub the fish with dried thyme, and ground black pepper.
2. Then fill the fish with sliced lemon and sprinkle with olive oil.
3. Place the trout in the slow cooker and add water.
4. Cook the fish on Low for 5 hours.

Nutritional info per serve: 252 calories, 30.4g protein, 1.9g carbohydrates, 13.2g fat, 0.6g fiber, 84mg cholesterol, 368mg sodium, 554mg potassium.

Braised Salmon

Yield: 4 servings | **Prep time:** 10 minutes | **Cook time:** 1 hour

Ingredients:

- 1 cup of water
- 2-pound salmon fillet
- 1 teaspoon ground black pepper

Method:

1. Put all ingredients in the slow cooker and close the lid.
2. Cook the salmon on High for 1 hour.

Nutritional info per serve: 301 calories, 44.1g protein, 0.3g carbohydrates, 14g fat, 0.1g fiber, 100mg cholesterol, 683mg sodium, 878mg potassium.

Seabass Ragout

Yield: 4 servings | **Prep time:** 15 minutes | **Cook time:** 3.5 hours

Ingredients:

- 7 oz shiitake mushrooms
- 1 yellow onion, diced
- 1 tablespoon coconut oil
- 1 teaspoon ground coriander
- 1 cup of water
- 12 oz seabass fillet, chopped

Method:

1. Heat the coconut oil in the skillet.
2. Add onion and mushrooms and roast the vegetables for 5 minutes on medium heat.
3. Then transfer the vegetables to the slow cooker and add water.
4. Add fish fillet, and ground coriander.
5. Cook the meal on High for 3.5 hours.

Nutritional info per serve: 241 calories, 20.4g protein, 9.4g carbohydrates, 14g fat, 2.3g fiber, 0mg cholesterol, 413mg sodium, 99mg potassium.

Shrimps with Cheese

Prep time: 10 minutes | **Cook time:** 5 minutes | **Yield:** 4 servings

Ingredients:

- 1-pound shrimps, peeled
- ½ cup almond flour
- 1 tablespoon olive oil
- 1 tablespoon mascarpone cheese

Method:

1. Dip the shrimps in the mascarpone cheese and coat in the almond flour.
2. Heat the olive oil in the slow cooker on saute mode for 2 minutes.
3. Put the coated shrimps in the slow cooker and cook them on saute mode for 1.5 minutes from each side.

Nutritional info per serve: 192 calories, 27g protein, 2.6g carbohydrates, 7.7g fat, 0.4g fiber, 241mg cholesterol, 281mg sodium, 196mg potassium.

Apple Cider Vinegar Mussels

Prep time: 10 minutes | **Cook time:** 5 minutes | **Yield:** 6 servings

Ingredients:

- 18 oz mussels, fresh
- 1 cup apple cider vinegar
- 1 teaspoon coconut
- oil, melted
- ¼ cup of water
- 1 teaspoon minced garlic

Method:

1. Pour water and apple cider vinegar into the slow cooker.
2. Then insert the steamer rack.
3. Put the mussels in the slow cooker mold.
4. Sprinkle them with coconut oil and minced garlic.
5. Close and seal the lid.
6. Cook the seafood on manual (high pressure) for 3 minutes. Make a quick pressure release.
7. If the mussels are not opened, cook them 2 minutes extra.

Nutritional info per serve: 89 calories, 10.2g protein, 3.7g carbohydrates, 2.7g fat, 0g fiber, 24mg cholesterol, 246mg sodium, 303mg potassium.

Salmon Caprese

Prep time: 10 minutes | **Cook time:** 15 minutes | **Yield:** 3 servings

Ingredients:

- 10 oz salmon fillet (2 fillets)
- 4 oz Mozzarella, sliced
- 4 cherry tomatoes, sliced
- 1 teaspoon Erythritol
- 1 teaspoon dried basil
- ½ teaspoon ground black pepper
- 1 tablespoon apple cider vinegar
- 1 tablespoon coconut oil
- 1 cup water, for cooking

Method:

1. Grease the mold with coconut oil and put the salmon inside.
2. Sprinkle the fish with Erythritol, dried basil, ground black pepper, and apple cider vinegar.
3. Then top the salmon with tomatoes and Mozzarella.
4. Pour water and insert the steamer rack into the slow cooker.
5. Put the fish on the rack.
6. Close and seal the lid.
7. Cook the meal on manual mode (high pressure0 for 15 minutes. Make a quick pressure release.

Nutritional info per serve: 302 calories, 30.5g protein, 9.7g carbohydrates, 17.4g fat, 2.1g fiber, 62mg cholesterol, 277mg sodium, 760mg potassium.

Thyme Lobster Tails

Prep time: 10 minutes | **Cook time:** 4 minutes | **Yield:** 4 servings

Ingredients:
- 4 lobster tails
- 1 tablespoon butter, softened
- 1 teaspoon dry thyme
- 1 cup of water

Method:
1. Pour water and insert the steamer rack into the slow cooker.
2. Put the lobster tails on the rack and close the lid.
3. Cook the meal on manual mode (high pressure) for 4 minutes. Make a quick pressure release.
4. After this, mix up butter and dry thyme.
5. Peel the lobsters and rub them with thyme butter.

Nutritional info per serve: 102 calories, 16.2g protein, 0.2g carbohydrates, 3.6g fat, 0.1g fiber, 132mg cholesterol, 435mg sodium, 199mg potassium.

Blackened Salmon

Prep time: 10 minutes | **Cook time:** 4 minutes | **Yield:** 3 servings

Ingredients:
- 1-pound salmon fillet
- 1 teaspoon ground black pepper
- 1 teaspoon ground turmeric
- 1 teaspoon lemon juice
- 1 cup of water

Method:
1. In the shallow bowl, mix up ground black pepper and ground turmeric.
2. Sprinkle the salmon fillet with lemon juice and rub with the spice mixture.
3. Then pour water into the slow cooker and insert the steamer rack.
4. Wrap the salmon fillet in the foil and place it on the rack.
5. Close and seal the lid.
6. Cook the fish on manual mode (high pressure) for 4 minutes.
7. Make a quick pressure release and cut the fish on servings.

Nutritional info per serve: 205 calories, 29.5g protein, 1g carbohydrates, 9.4g fat, 0.4g fiber, 67mg cholesterol, 70mg sodium, 611mg potassium.

Shrimp Curry with Coconut Milk

Prep time: 10 minutes | **Cook time:** 4 minutes | **Yield:** 5 servings

Ingredients:
- 15 oz shrimps, peeled
- 1 teaspoon chili powder
- 1 teaspoon garam masala
- 1 cup of coconut milk
- 1 teaspoon olive oil
- ½ teaspoon minced garlic

Method:
1. Heat the slow cooker on saute mode for 2 minutes.
2. Then add olive oil. Cook the ingredients for 1 minute.
3. Add shrimps and sprinkle them with chili powder, garam masala, minced garlic, and coconut milk.
4. Carefully stir the ingredients and close the lid.
5. Cook the shrimp curry on manual mode for 1 minute. Make a quick pressure release.

Nutritional info per serve: 222 calories, 20.6g protein, 4.3g carbohydrates, 13.9g fat, 1.3g fiber, 179mg cholesterol, 221mg sodium, 281mg potassium.

Spicy Cod

Prep time: 10 minutes | **Cook time:** 10 minutes | **Yield:** 2 servings

Ingredients:
- 2 cod fillet
- ¼ teaspoon chili powder
- ½ teaspoon cayenne pepper
- ½ teaspoon dried oregano
- 1 tablespoon lime juice
- 2 tablespoons avocado oil

Method:
1. Rub the cod fillets with chili powder, cayenne pepper, dried oregano, and sprinkle with lime juice.
2. Then pour the avocado oil into the slow cooker and heat it on saute mode for 2 minutes.
3. Put the cod fillets in the hot oil and cook for 5 minutes.
4. Then flip the fish on another side and cook for 5 minutes more.

Nutritional info per serve: 112 calories, 20.3g protein, 1.5g carbohydrates, 3g fat, 1g fiber, 55mg cholesterol, 74mg sodium, 66mg potassium.

Shrimp Skewers

Prep time: 10 minutes | **Cook time:** 2 minutes | **Yield:** 4 servings

Ingredients:

- 1 tablespoon lemon juice
- 1 teaspoon coconut aminos
- 12 oz shrimps, peeled
- 1 teaspoon olive oil
- 1 cup of water

Method:

1. Put the shrimps in the mixing bowl.
2. Add lemon juice, coconut aminos, and olive oil.
3. Then string the shrimps on the skewers.
4. Pour water into the slow cooker.
5. Then insert the trivet.
6. Put the shrimp skewers on the trivet.
7. Close the lid and cook the seafood on manual mode (high pressure) for 2 minutes.
8. When the time is finished, make a quick pressure release.

Nutritional info per serve: 113 calories, 19.4g protein, 1.6g carbohydrates, 2.6g fat, 0g fiber, 179mg cholesterol, 211mg sodium, 149mg potassium.

Salmon Cakes

Prep time: 15 minutes | **Cook time:** 10 minutes | **Yield:** 4 servings

Ingredients:

- 1-pound salmon fillet, chopped
- 1 tablespoon dill, chopped
- 2 eggs, beaten
- ½ cup almond flour
- 1 tablespoon coconut oil

Method:

1. Put the chopped salmon, dill, eggs, and almond flour in the food processor.
2. Blend the mixture until it is smooth.
3. Then make the small balls (cakes) from the salmon mixture.
4. After this, heat the coconut oil on saute mode for 3 minutes.
5. Put the salmon cakes in the slow cooker in one layer and cook them on saute mode for 2 minutes from each side or until they are light brown.

Nutritional info per serve: 297 calories, 27.9g protein, 3.6g carbohydrates, 19.3g fat, 1.6g fiber, 132mg cholesterol, 87mg sodium, 491mg potassium.

Lime Mahi Mahi

Prep time: 10 minutes | **Cook time:** 9 minutes | **Yield:** 4 servings

Ingredients:

- 1-pound mahi-mahi fillet
- 1 teaspoon lemon zest, grated
- 1 tablespoon lemon
- juice
- 1 tablespoon butter, softened
- 1 cup water, for cooking

Method:

1. Cut the fish into 4 servings and sprinkle with lemon zest, lemon juice, and rub with softened butter.
2. Then put the fish in the baking pan in one layer.
3. Pour water and insert the steamer rack into the slow cooker.
4. Put the mold with fish on the rack. Close and seal the lid.
5. Cook the Mahi Mahi on manual mode (high pressure) for 9 minutes. Make a quick pressure release.

Nutritional info per serve: 117 calories, 21.1g protein, 0.2g carbohydrates, 2.9g fat, 0.1g fiber, 48mg cholesterol, 117mg sodium, 7mg potassium.

Pesto Flounder

Prep time: 15 minutes | **Cook time:** 15 minutes | **Yield:** 3 servings

Ingredients:

- 2 tablespoons keto pesto sauce
- ½ cup coconut oil
- 10 oz flounder fillet
- 1 cup water, for cooking

Method:

1. Cut the fish into 3 servings and put it in the baking pan.
2. Brush the flounder fillets with pesto sauce. Add coconut oil.
3. Pour water and insert the steamer rack into the slow cooker.
4. Put the baking pan with fish on the rack. Close and seal the lid.
5. Cook the meal on manual mode (high pressure) for 15 minutes. Allow the natural pressure release for 10 minutes.

Nutritional info per serve: 455 calories, 23.5g protein, 0.3g carbohydrates, 40.8g fat, 0g fiber, 66mg cholesterol, 159mg sodium, 325mg potassium.

Alaskan Crab Legs

Prep time: 10 minutes | **Cook time:** 4 minutes | **Yield:** 4 servings

Ingredients:

- 1-pound Alaskan crab legs
- 1 tablespoon butter
- ¼ teaspoon dried cilantro
- 1 cup of water

Method:

1. Pour water into the slow cooker.
2. Add dried cilantro and crab legs.
3. Cook the on manual mode (high pressure) for 4 minutes.
4. Then make a quick pressure release.
5. Peel the crab legs and sprinkle them with butter.

Nutritional info per serve: 31 calories, 4.8g protein, 0.1g carbohydrates, 1.3g fat, 0.1g fiber, 14mg cholesterol, 227mg sodium, 1mg potassium.

Spinach Tuna Cakes

Prep time: 15 minutes | **Cook time:** 8 minutes | **Yield:** 4 servings

Ingredients:

- 10 oz tuna, grinded
- 1 cup spinach
- 1 egg, beaten
- 1 teaspoon ground
- coriander
- 2 tablespoon coconut flakes
- 1 tablespoon avocado oil

Method:

1. Blend the spinach in the blender until smooth.
2. Then transfer it to the mixing bowl and add grinded tuna, egg, and ground coriander.
3. Add coconut flakes and stir the mass with the help of the spoon.
4. Heat avocado oil in the slow cooker on saute mode for 2 minutes.
5. Then make the medium size cakes from the tuna mixture and place them in the hot oil.
6. Cook the tuna cakes on saute mode for 3 minutes.
7. Then flip the on another side and cook for 3 minutes more or until they are light brown.

Nutritional info per serve: 163 calories, 20.5g protein, 0.9g carbohydrates, 8.1g fat, 0.6g fiber, 63mg cholesterol, 57mg sodium, 313mg potassium.

Rosemary Catfish Steak

Prep time: 10 minutes | **Cook time:** 20 minutes | **Yield:** 4 servings

Ingredients:

- 16 oz catfish fillet
- 1 tablespoon dried rosemary
- 1 teaspoon garlic powder
- 1 tablespoon avocado oil
- 1 cup water, for cooking

Method:

1. Cut the catfish fillet into 4 steaks.
2. Then sprinkle them with dried rosemary, garlic powder, and avocado oil.
3. Place the fish steak in the baking mold in one layer.
4. After this, pour water and insert the steamer rack into the slow cooker.
5. Put the baking mold with fish on the rack. Close and seal the lid.
6. Cook the meal on manual (high pressure) for 20 minutes. Make a quick pressure release.

Nutritional info per serve: 163 calories, 17.8g protein, g c1.2arbohydrates, 9.2g fat, 0.6g fiber, 53mg cholesterol, 61mg sodium, 391mg potassium.

Louisiana Gumbo

Prep time: 10 minutes | **Cook time:** 4 minutes | **Yield:** 6 servings

Ingredients:

- 1-pound shrimps
- ¼ cup celery stalk, chopped
- 1 chili pepper, chopped
- ¼ cup okra, chopped
- 1 tablespoon coconut oil
- 2 cups chicken broth
- 1 teaspoon keto tomato paste

Method:

1. Put all ingredients in the slow cooker and stir until you get a light red color.
2. Then close and seal the lid.
3. Cook the meal on manual mode (high pressure) for 4 minutes.
4. When the time is finished, allow the natural pressure release for 10 minutes.

Nutritional info per serve: 126 calories, 19g protein, 2.1g carbohydrates, 4g fat, 0.3g fiber, 159mg cholesterol, 443mg sodium, 231mg potassium.

Lemon Salmon

Prep time: 10 minutes | **Cook time:** 4 minutes | **Yield:** 4 servings

Ingredients:

- 1-pound salmon fillet
- 1 tablespoon butter, melted
- 2 tablespoons lemon juice
- 1 teaspoon dried dill
- 1 cup of water

Method:

1. Cut the salmon fillet into 4 servings.
2. Line the slow cooker baking pan with foil and put the salmon fillets inside in one layer.
3. Then sprinkle the fish with dried dill, lemon juice, and butter.
4. Pour water into the slow cooker and insert the rack.
5. Place the baking pan with salmon on the rack and close the lid.
6. Cook the meal on manual mode (high pressure) for 4 minutes. Allow the natural pressure release for 5 minutes and remove the fish from the slow cooker.

Nutritional info per serve: 178 calories, 22.1g protein, 0.3g carbohydrates, 10g fat, 0.1g fiber, 58mg cholesterol, 74mg sodium, 455mg potassium.

Chili Haddock

Prep time: 10 minutes | **Cook time:** 5 minutes | **Yield:** 4 servings

Ingredients:

- 1 chili pepper, minced
- 1-pound haddock, chopped
- ½ teaspoon ground turmeric
- ½ cup fish stock
- 1 cup of water

Method:

1. In the mixing bowl mix up chili pepper, ground turmeric, and fish stock.
2. Then add chopped haddock and transfer the mixture to the baking mold.
3. Pour water into the slow cooker and insert the trivet.
4. Place the baking mold with fish on the trivet and close the lid.
5. Cook the meal on manual (high pressure) for 5 minutes. Make a quick pressure release.

Nutritional info per serve: 133 calories, 28.2g protein, 0.3g carbohydrates, 1.2g fat, 0.1g fiber, 84mg cholesterol, 146mg sodium, 505mg potassium.

Boiled Crawfish

Prep time: 5 minutes | **Cook time:** 5 minutes | **Yield:** 4 servings

Ingredients:

- 16 oz crawfish
- 1 teaspoon old bay
- seasonings
- 1 cup of water

Method:

1. Pour water into the slow cooker bowl.
2. Add old bay seasonings and crawfish.
3. Close and seal the lid and cook the seafood on manual mode (high pressure) for 5 minutes.
4. Then make a quick pressure release and transfer the cooked crawfish to the plate.

Nutritional info per serve: 99 calories, 19.9g protein, 0g carbohydrates, 1.5g fat, 0g fiber, 155mg cholesterol, 272mg sodium, 270mg potassium.

Pulpo Gallego

Prep time: 10 minutes | **Cook time:** 15 minutes | **Yield:** 4 servings

Ingredients:

- 1-pound octopus, rinsed
- 1 garlic clove, diced
- 1 tablespoon coconut oil, melted
- 1 cup of water

Method:

1. Put the octopus in the slow cooker.
2. Add coconut oil and diced garlic. Mix up the ingredients and add water.
3. Close and seal the lid.
4. Cook the meal on manual mode (high pressure) for 15 minutes.
5. Then allow the natural pressure release for 10 minutes.
6. Transfer the cooked octopus to the serving plate.

Nutritional info per serve: 216 calories, 33.9g protein, 5.2g carbohydrates, 5.8g fat, 0g fiber, 109mg cholesterol, 524mg sodium, 718mg potassium.

Clam Chowder

Prep time: 10 minutes | **Cook time:** 4 minutes | **Yield:** 2 servings

Ingredients:

- 5 oz clams
- 1 oz bacon, chopped
- 3 oz celery, chopped
- ½ cup of water
- ½ cup coconut cream

Method:

1. Cook the bacon on saute mode for 1 minute.
2. Then add clams, celery, water, and coconut cream.
3. Close and seal the lid.
4. Cook the seafood on steam mode (high pressure) for 3 minutes. Make a quick pressure release.
5. Ladle the clams with the heavy cream mixture in the bowls.

Nutritional info per serve: 255 calories, 7.3g protein, 12.5g carbohydrates, 20.4g fat, 2.3g fiber, 16mg cholesterol, 629mg sodium, 412mg potassium.

Italian Style Salmon

Prep time: 10 minutes | **Cook time:** 4 minutes | **Yield:** 2 servings

Ingredients:
- 10 oz salmon fillet
- 1 teaspoon Italian
- seasonings
- 1 cup of water

Method:

1. Pour water and insert the trivet in the slow cooker.
2. Then rub the salmon fillet with Italian seasonings and wrap it in the foil.
3. Place the wrapped fish on the trivet and close the lid.
4. Cook the meal on manual mode (high pressure) for 4 minutes.
5. Make a quick pressure release and remove the fish from the foil.
6. Cut it into servings.

Nutritional info per serve: 195 calories, 27.5g protein, 0.3g carbohydrates, 9.5g fat, 0g fiber, 64mg cholesterol, 67mg sodium, 547mg potassium.

Butter Clams

Prep time: 10 minutes | **Cook time:** 3 minutes | **Yield:** 2 servings

Ingredients:
- 7 oz clams
- 2 tablespoons butter
- 1 cup of water
- 1 teaspoon minced garlic

Method:

1. Pour water into the slow cooker.
2. Add clams and close the lid.
3. Cook the cams on high pressure for 3 minutes.

4. When the time is over, make a quick pressure release and transfer the hot clams to the bowl.
5. Add butter and minced garlic.
6. Shake the seafood well.

Nutritional info per serve: 152 calories, 0.8g protein, 11.3g carbohydrates, 11.7g fat, 0.4g fiber, 31mg cholesterol, 445mg sodium, 99mg potassium.

Cajun Cod

Prep time: 10 minutes | **Cook time:** 4 minutes | **Yield:** 2 servings

Ingredients:
- 10 oz cod fillet
- 1 tablespoon olive oil
- 1 teaspoon Cajun
- seasonings
- 2 tablespoons coconut aminos

Method:

1. Sprinkle the cod fillet with coconut aminos and Cajun seasonings.
2. Then heat olive oil in the slow cooker on saute mode.
3. Add the spiced cod fillet and cook it for 4 minutes from each side.
4. Then cut it into halves and sprinkle with the oily liquid from the slow cooker.

Nutritional info per serve: 189 calories, 25.3g protein, 3g carbohydrates, 8.3g fat, 0g fiber, 70mg cholesterol, 131mg sodium, 0mg potassium.

Fish Curry

Prep time: 10 minutes | **Cook time:** 3 minutes | **Yield:** 2 servings

Ingredients:
- 8 oz cod fillet, chopped
- 1 teaspoon curry
- paste
- 1 cup organic almond milk

Method:

1. Mix up curry paste and almond milk and pour the liquid into the slow cooker.
2. Add chopped cod fillet and close the lid.
3. Cook the fish curry on manual mode (high pressure) for 3 minutes.
4. Then make the quick pressure release for 5 minutes.

Nutritional info per serve: 384 calories, 24.1g protein, 7.4g carbohydrates, 31.1g fat, 2.6g fiber, 56mg cholesterol, 89mg sodium, 316mg potassium.

Seafood Zoodle Alfredo

Prep time: 10 minutes | **Cook time:** 10 minutes | **Yield:** 4 servings

Ingredients:

- 2 zucchinis, trimmed
- 1 cup coconut milk
- 1 teaspoon coconut oil
- 1 teaspoon seafood seasonings
- 6 oz shrimps, peeled

Method:

1. Melt the coconut oil on saute mode and add shrimps.

2. Sprinkle them with seafood seasonings and saute them for 2 minutes.

3. After this, spiralizer the zucchini with the help of the spiralizer and add in the shrimps.

4. Add coconut milk and close the lid. Cook the meal on saute mode for 8 minutes.

Nutritional info per serve: 214 calories, 12.2g protein, 7.3g carbohydrates, 16.3g fat, 2.4g fiber, 90mg cholesterol, 123mg sodium, 487mg potassium.

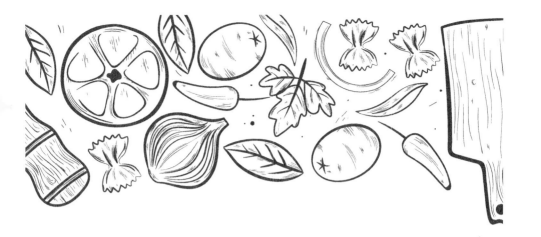

Soups and Stews

Broccoli Cheese Soup

Prep time: 10 minutes | **Cook time:** 5 minutes | **Yield:** 4 servings

Ingredients:

- 2 cups broccoli florets
- 1 cup Cheddar cheese, shredded
- 2 garlic cloves, diced
- 1 tablespoon olive oil
- 1 cup coconut cream
- 2 cups chicken broth
- ½ teaspoon ground black pepper

Method:

1. Heat olive oil in the slow cooker.
2. Then add diced garlic and saute it for 2 minutes.
3. After this, add broccoli florets, shredded cheese, coconut cream, and chicken broth.
4. Add ground black pepper and close the lid.
5. Cook the soup on manual mode (High pressure) for 3 minutes.
6. Then allow the natural pressure release for 5 minutes.

Nutritional info per serve: 319 calories, 12.2g protein, 7.8g carbohydrates, 28g fat, 2.6g fiber, 30mg cholesterol, 581mg sodium, 442mg potassium.

Gumbo

Prep time: 10 minutes | **Cook time:** 15 minutes | **Yield:** 4 servings

Ingredients:

- 2 chicken thighs, boneless, chopped
- 4 oz shrimps, peeled
- ½ bell pepper, chopped
- 3 oz sausages, chopped, homemade
- 1 celery stalk, chopped
- 1 cup beef broth
- 1 teaspoon keto tomato paste
- ½ teaspoon Cajun seasonings

Method:

1. Heat the slow cooker on saute mode for 3 minutes.
2. Then add chicken thighs, shrimps, bell pepper, sausages, celery stalk, beef broth, tomato paste, and Cajun seasonings.
3. Gently mix up the ingredients and close the lid.
4. Cook the gumbo for 15 minutes on manual mode (high pressure).
5. Then make a quick pressure release and stir the meal well.

Nutritional info per serve: 261 calories, 33.2g protein, 2.2g carbohydrates, 12.3g fat, 0.4g fiber, 143mg cholesterol, 493mg sodium, 392mg potassium.

Chicken Soup

Prep time: 10 minutes | **Cook time:** 20 minutes | **Yield:** 2 servings

Ingredients:

- 8 oz chicken breast, skinless, boneless
- 2 cups of water
- 1 tablespoon
- scallions, diced
- 1 tablespoon fresh dill, chopped

Method:

1. Pour water into the slow cooker.
2. Chop the chicken breast and add it to the water.
3. Then add scallions, and close the lid.
4. Cook the soup on manual mode (high pressure) for 20 minutes.
5. Then make a quick pressure release.
6. Top the cooked soup with fresh dill.

Nutritional info per serve: 134 calories, 24.4g protein, 1.1g carbohydrates, 2.9g fat, 0.3g fiber, 73mg cholesterol, 69mg sodium, 482mg potassium.

Taco Soup

Prep time: 15 minutes | **Cook time:** 20 minutes | **Yield:** 6 servings

Ingredients:

- 1 cup ground beef
- 1 bell pepper, chopped
- 1 garlic clove, diced
- ¼ cup crushed tomatoes
- 2 tablespoons cream cheese
- 4 cups beef broth
- 1 tablespoon coconut oil
- 1 teaspoon taco seasonings

Method:

1. Heat coconut oil in the slow cooker on saute mode.
2. Then add ground beef and sprinkle it with taco seasonings. Stir well and cook the meat on saute mode for 5 minutes.
3. After this, add bell pepper, garlic clove, crushed tomatoes, cream cheese, and beef broth.
4. Close the lid and cook the soup on manual mode (high pressure) for 15 minutes.
5. Then allow the natural pressure release for 10 minutes and open the lid.
6. Ladle the soup.

Nutritional info per serve: 103 calories, 7.5g protein, 3.5g carbohydrates, 6.4g fat, 0.6g fiber, 16mg cholesterol, 585mg sodium, 181mg potassium.

Tuscan Soup

Prep time: 15 minutes | **Cook time:** 13 minutes | **Yield:** 3 servings

Ingredients:

- 1 bacon slice, chopped
- 2 oz scallions, diced
- ½ teaspoon garlic powder
- 6 oz Italian sausages, chopped
- ¼ cup cauliflower, chopped
- 3 cups chicken broth
- 1 cup kale, chopped
- ¼ cup coconut cream

Method:

1. Heat the slow cooker on saute mode for 3 minutes.
2. Then add chopped bacon and cook it for 2 minutes on saute mode.
3. Stir it well and add scallions.
4. Add garlic powder, Italian sausages, and cauliflower.
5. Mix up the ingredients and cook them for 5 minutes on saute mode.
6. After this, add chicken broth, kale, and coconut cream.
7. Cook the soup on manual mode (high pressure) for 6 minutes. Then make a quick pressure release.

Nutritional info per serve: 336 calories, 17g protein, 7g carbohydrates, 26.6g fat, 1.5g fiber, 50mg cholesterol, 134mg sodium, 630mg potassium.

Beef Stew

Prep time: 10 minutes | **Cook time:** 30 minutes | **Yield:** 4 servings

Ingredients:

- ½ cup Brussel sprouts
- 4 cups of water
- 1 teaspoon keto tomato paste
- 12 oz beef sirloin, chopped
- 1 tablespoon avocado oil
- 1 bay leaf
- ½ teaspoon peppercorns

Method:

1. Put all ingredients in the slow cooker and close the lid.
2. Cook the stew on Manual mode (high pressure) for 30 minutes.
3. The cooked stew should have a very tender structure.

Nutritional info per serve: 170 calories, 26.3g protein, 1.8g carbohydrates, 5.8g fat, 0.8g fiber, 76mg cholesterol, 67mg sodium, 417mg potassium.

Cheeseburger Soup

Prep time: 10 minutes | **Cook time:** 11 minutes | **Yield:** 5 servings

Ingredients:

- 1 cup ground pork
- 1 teaspoon mustard powder
- 4 cups beef broth
- 1 teaspoon cayenne pepper
- 1 teaspoon coconut
- oil
- ½ cup Monterey jack cheese, shredded
- 2 tablespoons cream cheese
- 3 tablespoons coconut cream

Method:

1. In the mixing bowl, mix up ground pork, mustard powder, and cayenne pepper.
2. Then melt the coconut oil in the slow cooker on saute mode.
3. Add the ground pork mixture and saute it for 6 minutes.
4. Then stir the mixture well and add cream cheese and coconut cream. Add beef broth and close the lid.
5. Cook the soup on manual mode (high pressure) for 5 minutes.
6. Then make a quick pressure release and ladle the soup in the bowls.
7. Top the soup with Monterey Jack cheese.

Nutritional info per serve: 170 calories, 11.8g protein, 1.9g carbohydrates, 12.8g fat, 0.4g fiber, 30mg cholesterol, 696mg sodium, 214mg potassium.

Cabbage Soup

Prep time: 10 minutes | **Cook time:** 12 minutes | **Yield:** 3 servings

Ingredients:

- ½ cup ground pork
- ½ cup white cabbage, shredded
- 2 cups chicken broth
- ½ teaspoon ground coriander
- 1 teaspoon butter
- ½ teaspoon chili flakes

Method:

1. Melt the butter in the slow cooker on saute mode.
2. Add cabbage and sprinkle it with ground coriander, and chili flakes.
3. Add chicken broth and ground pork.
4. Close and seal the lid and cook the soup on manual mode (high pressure) for 12 minutes.

Nutritional info per serve: 108 calories, 9.1g protein, 1.3g carbohydrates, 7.2g fat, 0.3g fiber, 3mg cholesterol, 520mg sodium, 159mg potassium.

Cauliflower Soup

Prep time: 15 minutes | **Cook time:** 6 minutes | **Yield:** 4 servings

Ingredients:

- 2 cups cauliflower, chopped
- 1 cup coconut cream
- 2 cups beef broth
- 2 tablespoons fresh cilantro
- 3 oz Provolone cheese, chopped

Method:

1. Put cauliflower, coconut cream, beef broth, cilantro, and cheese in the slow cooker.
2. Cook the soup on manual (high pressure) for 6 minutes. Then allow the natural pressure release for 4 minutes.
3. Blend the soup with the help of the immersion blender.

Nutritional info per serve: 244 calories, 10.2g protein, 6.9g carbohydrates, 20.7g fat, 2.6g fiber, 15mg cholesterol, 592mg sodium, 444mg potassium.

Chicken Paprikash

Prep time: 10 minutes | **Cook time:** 18 minutes | **Yield:** 4 servings

Ingredients:

- 1 tablespoon ground paprika
- ¼ cup scallions, diced
- 1 bell pepper, chopped
- 4 chicken thighs, skinless
- 1 teaspoon coconut oil
- ½ teaspoon ground cumin
- 4 cups chicken broth

Method:

1. Heat coconut oil in the slow cooker on Saute mode.
2. When the oil is melted. Add chicken thighs and cook them for 4 minutes from each side.
3. After this, sprinkle the chicken scallions, bell pepper, and ground cumin. Gently mix up the ingredients. Add paprika.
4. Add chicken broth and close the lid.
5. Cook the paprikash for 10 minutes on Manual mode (high pressure). Then make a quick pressure release.

Nutritional info per serve: 343 calories, 47.8g protein, 4.7g carbohydrates, 13.7g fat, 1.2g fiber, 130mg cholesterol, 892mg sodium, 680mg potassium.

Pork Stew

Prep time: 15 minutes | **Cook time:** 3 minutes | **Yield:** 6 servings

Ingredients:

- ½ cup daikon, chopped
- 1 oz green onions, chopped
- 1-pound pork tenderloin, chopped
- 1 lemon slice
- 1 teaspoon ground black pepper
- 1 tablespoon butter
- 1 tablespoon heavy cream
- 3 cups of water

Method:

1. Put all ingredients in the slow cooker and mix up them with the help of the spatula.
2. Then close and seal the lid. Set manual mode (high pressure) and cook the stew for 20 minutes.
3. Allow the natural pressure release for 15 minutes.

Nutritional info per serve: 137 calories, 20.1g protein, 0.9g carbohydrates, 5.5g fat, 0.3g fiber, 64mg cholesterol, 63mg sodium, 351mg potassium.

Curry Stew with Chicken

Prep time: 10 minutes | **Cook time:** 12 minutes | **Yield:** 4 servings

Ingredients:

- 1 teaspoon curry paste
- 1 teaspoon grated lemon zest
- 4 oz leek, chopped
- 2 cups of water
- 1 tablespoon coconut cream
- 4 chicken thighs, skinless, boneless, chopped

Method:

1. In the mixing bowl, mix up coconut cream, grated lemon zest, and curry paste.
2. Then mix up chopped chicken thighs and curry paste mixture.
3. Put the mixture in the slow cooker and add leek and water.
4. Close the lid and cook the stew for 12 minutes on manual mode (high pressure).
5. Then make a quick pressure release and transfer the stew to the plates/bowls.

Nutritional info per serve: 312 calories, 42.8g protein, 4.7g carbohydrates, 12.5g fat, 0.6g fiber, 130mg cholesterol, 135mg sodium, 418mg potassium.

Italian Style Lamb Stew

Prep time: 10 minutes | **Cook time:** 52 minutes | **Yield:** 5 servings

Ingredients:

- 1-pound lamb shank, chopped
- 1 teaspoon dried rosemary
- 1 turnip, chopped
- 1 teaspoon keto tomato paste
- 1 teaspoon olive oil
- 2 cups of water

Method:

1. Heat olive oil on saute mode for 2 minutes.
2. Then add turnip, chopped lamb shank, and dried rosemary. Saute the ingredients for 5 minutes.
3. After this, add water and tomato paste. Close the lid and cook the stew on saute mode for 45 minutes.

Nutritional info per serve: 185 calories, 25.8g protein, 1.9g carbohydrates, 7.7g fat, 0.6g fiber, 82mg cholesterol, 89mg sodium, 365mg potassium.

Cheesy Cream Soup

Prep time: 15 minutes | **Cook time:** 20 minutes | **Yield:** 4 servings

Ingredients:

- 3 tablespoons cream cheese
- 2 oz blue cheese, crumbled
- 2 cups white mushrooms, chopped
- 4 oz scallions, diced
- 4 cups chicken broth
- 1 teaspoon olive oil
- ½ teaspoon ground cumin

Method:

1. Put cream cheese, mushrooms, scallions, chicken broth, olive oil, and ground cumin in the slow cooker.
2. Close and seal the lid.
3. Cook the soup mixture for 20 minutes on manual mode (high pressure).
4. Then make a quick pressure release and open the lid.
5. Add salt and blend the soup with the help of the immersion blender.
6. Then ladle the soup in the bowls and top with blue cheese.

Nutritional info per serve: 142 calories, 10.1g protein, 4.8g carbohydrates, 9.4g fat, 1.1g fiber, 19mg cholesterol, 990mg sodium, 446mg potassium.

Seafood Stew

Prep time: 10 minutes | **Cook time:** 20 minutes | **Yield:** 4 servings

Ingredients:

- ½ teaspoon ground cumin
- ½ teaspoon ground paprika
- ½ teaspoon ground turmeric
- 8 oz cod, chopped
- 1 cup water
- 1 teaspoon coconut oil

Method:

1. Sprinkle the chopped cod with cumin, paprika, and turmeric.
2. Then heat coconut oil in the slow cooker on saute mode.
3. Add cod and cook it for 2 minutes from each side.
4. Then add water and close the lid.
5. Saute the stew for 15 minutes.

Nutritional info per serve: 72 calories, 13.1g protein, 0.4g carbohydrates, 1.7g fat, 0.2g fiber, 31mg cholesterol, 47mg sodium, 157mg potassium.

Keto Chili

Prep time: 10 minutes | **Cook time:** 25 minutes | **Yield:** 2 servings

Ingredients:

- ½ cup ground beef
- ½ teaspoon chili powder
- 1 teaspoon dried oregano
- ¼ cup apple cider vinegar
- 2 oz scallions, diced
- 1 teaspoon avocado oil
- ¼ cup of water

Method:

1. Mix up ground beef, chili powder, dried oregano, and scallions.
2. Then add avocado oil and stir the mixture.
3. Transfer it to the slow cooker and cook on saute mode for 10 minutes.
4. Add water and apple cider vinegar. Stir the ingredients with the help of the spatula until homogenous.
5. Close and seal the lid and cook the chili for 15 minutes on manual mode (high pressure). Then make a quick pressure release.

Nutritional info per serve: 132 calories, 12.5g protein, 3.3g carbohydrates, 7g fat, 1.4g fiber, 38mg cholesterol, 52mg sodium, 306mg potassium.

Okra and Beef Stew

Prep time: 15 minutes | **Cook time:** 25 minutes | **Yield:** 3 servings

Ingredients:

- 6 oz okra, chopped
- 8 oz beef sirloin, chopped
- 1 cup of water
- ¼ cup coconut milk
- 1 teaspoon dried basil
- ¼ teaspoon cumin seeds
- 1 tablespoon avocado oil

Method:

1. Sprinkle the beef sirloin with cumin seeds and dried basil and put it in the slow cooker.

2. Add avocado oil and roast the meat on saute mode for 5 minutes. Stir it occasionally.

3. Then add coconut milk, water, and okra.

4. Close the lid and cook the stew on manual mode (high pressure) for 25 minutes. Allow the natural pressure release for 10 minutes.

Nutritional info per serve: 216 calories, 24.6g protein, 5.7g carbohydrates, 10.2g fat, 2.5g fiber, 68mg cholesterol, 60mg sodium, 546mg potassium.

Chorizo Soup

Prep time: 10 minutes | **Cook time:** 17 minutes | **Yield:** 3 servings

Ingredients:

- 8 oz keto chorizo, chopped
- 1 teaspoon keto tomato paste
- 4 oz scallions, diced
- 1 tablespoon dried cilantro
- ½ teaspoon chili powder
- 1 teaspoon avocado oil
- 2 cups beef broth

Method:

1. Heat avocado oil on saute mode for 1 minute.

2. Add chorizo and cook it for 6 minutes, stir it from time to time.

3. Then add scallions, tomato paste, cilantro, and chili powder. Stir well.

4. Add beef broth.

5. Close and seal the lid.

6. Cook the soup on manual mode (high pressure) for 10 minutes. Make a quick pressure release.

Nutritional info per serve: 387 calories, 22.3g protein, 5.5g carbohydrates, 30.2g fat, 1.3g fiber, 67mg cholesterol, 145mg sodium, 576mg potassium.

Chipotle Stew

Prep time: 15 minutes | **Cook time:** 10 minutes | **Yield:** 3 servings

Ingredients:

- 2 chipotle chili, chopped
- 1 oz fresh cilantro, chopped
- 9 oz chicken fillet, chopped
- 1 teaspoon ground paprika
- 1 cup chicken broth

Method:

1. In the mixing bowl mix up chipotle chili, cilantro, chicken fillet, and ground paprika.

2. Then transfer the ingredients to the slow cooker and add chicken broth.

3. Cook the stew on manual mode (high pressure) for 10 minutes. Allow the natural pressure release for 10 minutes more.

Nutritional info per serve: 179 calories, 26.5g protein, 1g carbohydrates, 6.9g fat, 0.5g fiber, 76mg cholesterol, 332mg sodium, 341mg potassium.

Pizza Soup

Prep time: 10 minutes | **Cook time:** 22 minutes | **Yield:** 3 servings

Ingredients:

- ¼ cup cremini mushrooms, sliced
- 1 teaspoon keto tomato paste
- 4 oz Mozzarella, shredded
- ½ jalapeno pepper, sliced
- ½ teaspoon Italian seasoning
- 1 teaspoon coconut oil
- 5 oz keto Italian sausages, chopped
- 1 cup of water

Method:

1. Melt the coconut oil in the slow cooker on saute mode.

2. Add mushrooms and cook them for 10 minutes.

3. After this, add chopped sausages, Italian seasoning, sliced jalapeno, and tomato paste.

4. Mix up the ingredients well and add water.

5. Close and seal the lid and cook the soup on manual mode (high pressure) for 12 minutes.

6. Then make a quick pressure release and ladle the soup in the bowls. Top it with Mozzarella.

Nutritional info per serve: 289 calories, 19.9g protein, 4.2g carbohydrates, 21.3g fat, 0.3g fiber, 47mg cholesterol, 801mg sodium, 195mg potassium.

Lamb Soup

Prep time: 10 minutes | **Cook time:** 25 minutes | **Yield:** 4 servings

Ingredients:
- ½ cup broccoli, roughly chopped
- 7 oz lamb fillet, chopped
- ¼ teaspoon ground cumin
- ¼ daikon, chopped
- 2 bell peppers, chopped
- 1 tablespoon avocado oil
- 5 cups beef broth

Method:
1. Saute the lamb fillet with avocado oil in the slow cooker for 5 minutes.
2. Then add broccoli, ground cumin, daikon, bell peppers, and beef broth.
3. Close and seal the lid.
4. Cook the soup on manual mode (high pressure) for 20 minutes.
5. Allow the natural pressure release.

Nutritional info per serve: 169 calories, 21g protein, 6.8g carbohydrates, 6g fat, 1.3g fiber, 45mg cholesterol, 998mg sodium, 593mg potassium.

Minestrone Soup

Prep time: 10 minutes | **Cook time:** 25 minutes | **Yield:** 4 servings

Ingredients:
- 1 ½ cup ground pork
- ½ bell pepper, chopped
- 2 tablespoons chives, chopped
- 2 oz celery stalk, chopped
- 1 teaspoon coconut oil
- 1 teaspoon Italian seasonings
- 4 cups chicken broth
- ½ cup mushrooms, sliced

Method:
1. Heat the coconut oil on the saute mode for 2 minutes.
2. Add bell pepper. Cook the vegetable for 5 minutes.
3. Then stir them well and add mushrooms, celery stalk, and Italian seasonings. Stir well and cook for 5 minutes more.
4. Add ground pork, chives, and chicken broth.
5. Close and seal the lid.
6. Cook the soup on manual mode (high pressure) for 15 minutes. Make a quick pressure release.

Nutritional info per serve: 124 calories, 10.9g protein, 3g carbohydrates, 7.5g fat, 0.6g fiber, 21mg cholesterol, 791mg sodium, 304mg potassium.

Red Feta Soup

Prep time: 10 minutes | **Cook time:** 25 minutes | **Yield:** 4 servings

Ingredients:
- 1 cup broccoli, chopped
- 1 teaspoon keto tomato paste
- ½ cup coconut milk
- 4 cups beef broth
- 1 teaspoon chili flakes
- 6 oz plain feta, crumbled

Method:
1. Put broccoli, tomato paste, coconut cream, and beef broth in the slow cooker.
2. Add chili flakes and stir the mixture until it is red.
3. Then close and seal the lid and cook the soup for 8 minutes on manual mode (high pressure).
4. Then make a quick pressure release and open the lid.
5. Add feta cheese and saute the soup on saute mode for 5 minutes more.

Nutritional info per serve: 229 calories, 15g protein, 6.9g carbohydrates, 17.4g fat, 2.3g fiber, 31mg cholesterol, 126mg sodium, 372mg potassium.

"Ramen" Soup

Prep time: 10 minutes | **Cook time:** 15 minutes | **Yield:** 2 servings

Ingredients:
- 1 zucchini, trimmed
- 2 cups chicken broth
- 2 eggs, boiled, peeled
- 1 tablespoon coconut aminos
- 5 oz beef loin, strips
- 1 teaspoon chili flakes
- 1 tablespoon chives, chopped

Method:
1. Put the beef loin strips in the slow cooker.
2. Add chili flakes and chicken broth.
3. Close and seal the lid. Cook the ingredients on manual mode (high pressure) for 15 minutes. Make a quick pressure release and open the lid.
4. Then make the s from zucchini with the help of the spiralizer and add them to the soup.
5. Add chives and coconut aminos.
6. Then ladle the soup in the bowls and top with halved eggs.

Nutritional info per serve: 272 calories, 31.9g protein, 6.2g carbohydrates, 12.6g fat, 1.1g fiber, 218mg cholesterol, 891mg sodium, 809mg potassium.

Beef Tagine

Prep time: 15 minutes | **Cook time:** 25 minutes | **Yield:** 6 servings

Ingredients:

- 1-pound beef fillet, chopped
- 1 eggplant, chopped
- 6 oz scallions, chopped
- 1 teaspoon ground

allspices
- 1 teaspoon Erythritol
- 1 teaspoon coconut oil
- 4 cups beef broth

Method:

1. Put all ingredients in the slow cooker.
2. Close and seal the lid.
3. Cook the meal on manual mode (high pressure) for 25 minutes.
4. Then allow the natural pressure release for 15 minutes.

Nutritional info per serve: 198 calories, 24.7g protein, 8g carbohydrates, 8.2g fat, 3.4g fiber, 54mg cholesterol, 556mg sodium, 648mg potassium.

Yogurt Soup

Yield: 4 servings | **Prep time:** 10 minutes | **Cook time:** 5 hours

Ingredients:

- 1 cup Greek yogurt
- ½ teaspoon dried mint
- ½ teaspoon ground black pepper
- 1 onion, diced

- 1 tablespoon coconut oil
- 3 cups chicken stock
- 7 oz chicken fillet, chopped

Method:

1. Melt the coconut oil in the skillet.
2. Add onion and roast it until light brown.
3. After this, transfer the roasted onion to the slow cooker.
4. Add dried mint, ground black pepper, chicken stock, and chicken fillet.
5. Add Greek yogurt and carefully mix the soup ingredients.
6. Close the lid and cook the soup on High for 5 hours.

Nutritional info per serve: 180 calories, 20.2g protein, 5.3g carbohydrates, 8.6g fat, 0.7g fiber, 47mg cholesterol, 633mg sodium, 247mg potassium.

Chili Verde Soup

Prep time: 10 minutes | **Cook time:** 25 minutes | **Yield:** 4 servings

Ingredients:

- 2 oz keto chili Verde sauce
- ½ cup Cheddar cheese, shredded
- 5 cups chicken broth

- 1-pound chicken breast, skinless, boneless
- 1 tablespoon dried cilantro

Method:

1. Put chicken breast and chicken broth in the slow cooker.
2. Add cilantro, close, and seal the lid.
3. Then cook the ingredients on manual (high pressure) for 15 minutes.
4. Make a quick pressure release and open the li.
5. Shred the chicken breast with the help of the fork.
6. Add dried cilantro and chili Verde sauce to the soup and cook it on saute mode for 10 minutes.
7. Then add dried cilantro and stir well.

Nutritional info per serve: 234 calories, 33.6g protein, 1.3g carbohydrates, 9.2g fat, 0g fiber, 87mg cholesterol, 1100mg sodium, 693mg potassium.

Pepper Stuffing Soup

Prep time: 10 minutes | **Cook time:** 14 minutes | **Yield:** 4 servings

Ingredients:

- 1 cup ground beef
- ½ cup cauliflower, shredded
- 1 teaspoon dried oregano
- 1 teaspoon keto

tomato paste
- 1 teaspoon minced garlic
- 4 cups of water
- ¼ cup of coconut milk

Method:

1. Put all ingredients in the slow cooker bowl and stir well.
2. Then close and seal the lid.
3. Cook the soup on manual mode (high pressure) for 14 minutes.
4. When the time of cooking is finished, make a quick pressure release and open the lid.

Nutritional info per serve: 87 calories, 6.3g protein, 2.3g carbohydrates, 6.1g fat, 0.9g fiber, 18mg cholesterol, 29mg sodium, 173mg potassium.

Steak Soup

Prep time: 10 minutes | **Cook time:** 40 minutes | **Yield:** 5 servings

Ingredients:
- 5 oz scallions, diced
- 1 tablespoon coconut oil
- 1 oz daikon, diced
- 1-pound beef round steak, chopped
- 1 teaspoon dried thyme
- 5 cups of water
- ½ teaspoon ground black pepper

Method:
1. Heat coconut oil on saute mode for 2 minutes.
2. Add daikon and scallions.
3. After this, stir them well and add chopped beef steak, thyme, and ground black pepper.
4. Saute the ingredients for 5 minutes more and then add water.
5. Close and seal the lid.
6. Cook the soup on manual mode (high pressure) for 35 minutes. Make a quick pressure release.

Nutritional info per serve: 230 calories, 29.4g protein, 2.6g carbohydrates, 10.8g fat, 1g fiber, 76mg cholesterol, 68mg sodium, 499mg potassium.

Leek Soup

Prep time: 10 minutes | **Cook time:** 15 minutes | **Yield:** 4 servings

Ingredients:
- 7 oz leek, chopped
- 2 oz Monterey Jack cheese, shredded
- 1 teaspoon Italian seasonings
- 4 tablespoons coconut oil
- 2 cups chicken broth

Method:
1. Heat coconut oil in the slow cooker for 4 minutes.
2. Then add chopped leek and Italian seasonings.
3. Cook the leek on saute mode for 5 minutes. Stir the vegetables from time to time.
4. After this, add chicken broth and close the lid.
5. Cook the soup in saute mode for 10 minutes.
6. Then add shredded cheese and stir it till the cheese is melted.
7. The soup is cooked.

Nutritional info per serve: 223 calories, 6.6g protein, 7.7g carbohydrates, 19.1g fat, 0.9g fiber, 13mg cholesterol, 468mg sodium, 205mg potassium.

Asparagus Soup

Prep time: 10 minutes | **Cook time:** 17 minutes | **Yield:** 4 servings

Ingredients:
- 1 cup asparagus, chopped
- 2 cups of coconut milk
- ½ teaspoon cayenne pepper
- 3 oz scallions, diced
- 1 teaspoon olive oil

Method:
1. Saute the chopped asparagus, scallions, and olive oil in the slow cooker for 7 minutes.
2. Then stir the vegetables well and add cayenne pepper, and coconut milk
3. Cook the soup on manual mode (high pressure) for 10 minutes.
4. After this, make a quick pressure release and open the lid.
5. Blend the soup until you get the creamy texture.

Nutritional info per serve: 300 calories, 3.9g protein, 9.6g carbohydrates, 29.9g fat, 4g fiber, 0mg cholesterol, 22mg sodium, 447mg potassium.

Curry Kale Soup

Prep time: 10 minutes | **Cook time:** 15 minutes | **Yield:** 3 servings

Ingredients:
- 2 cups kale
- 1 tablespoon fresh cilantro
- 1 teaspoon curry paste
- ½ cup coconut milk
- ½ cup ground chicken
- 1 teaspoon coconut oil
- 1 cup chicken stock

Method:
1. Blend the kale until smooth and put it in the slow cooker.
2. Add cilantro, coconut oil, and ground chicken. Saute the mixture for 5 minutes.
3. Meanwhile, in the shallow bowl, mix up curry paste and coconut milk. When the liquid is smooth, pour it into the slow cooker.
4. Add chicken stock and close the lid.
5. Cook the soup on manual (high pressure) for 10 minutes. Make a quick pressure release.

Nutritional info per serve: 186 calories, 9.3g protein, 7.6g carbohydrates, 13.9g fat, 1.6g fiber, 21mg cholesterol, 300mg sodium, 388mg potassium.

Turmeric Rutabaga Soup

Prep time: 15 minutes | **Cook time:** 15 minutes | **Yield:** 6 servings

Ingredients:

- 3 turnips, chopped
- 1 teaspoon ginger paste
- 2 oz celery, chopped
- 1 teaspoon ground turmeric
- 1 teaspoon minced

- garlic
- 2 cups of coconut milk
- 1 cup beef broth
- 2 oz bell pepper, chopped

Method:

1. Place all ingredients in the slow cooker and stir them gently.
2. Then close and seal the lid; set manual mode (high pressure) and cook the soup for 15 minutes.
3. Then allow the natural pressure release for 10 minutes and ladle the soup into the serving bowls.

Nutritional info per serve: 225 calories, 3.7g protein, 12.5g carbohydrates, 19.5g fat, 3.6g fiber, 0mg cholesterol, 188mg sodium, 474mg potassium.

French Soup

Yield: 5 servings | **Prep time:** 10 minutes | **Cook time:** 7 hours

Ingredients:

- 5 oz Gruyere cheese, shredded
- 2 cups of water
- 2 cups chicken stock

- 2 cups white onion, diced
- ½ teaspoon cayenne pepper
- ½ cup heavy cream

Method:

1. Pour chicken stock, water, and heavy cream into the slow cooker.
2. Add onion, cayenne pepper, and close the lid.
3. Cook the ingredients on high for 4 hours.
4. When the time is finished, open the lid, stir the mixture, and add cheese.
5. Carefully mix the soup and cook it on Low for 3 hours.

Nutritional info per serve: 181 calories, 9.5g protein, 5.1g carbohydrates, 13.9g fat, 1g fiber, 48mg cholesterol, 410mg sodium, 110mg potassium.

Chicken and Noodles Soup

Yield: 8 servings | **Prep time:** 10 minutes | **Cook time:** 7 hours

Ingredients:

- 1-pound chicken breast, skinless, boneless, chopped
- 1 teaspoon chili flakes
- 1 teaspoon coriander

- 1 cup bell pepper, chopped
- 4 oz zucchini, spiralized
- 8 cups chicken stock

Method:

1. Mix chicken breast with salt, chili flakes, coriander, and place in the slow cooker.
2. Add chicken stock and close the lid.
3. Cook the ingredients on Low for 6 hours.
4. Then add spiralized zucchini and bell pepper and cook the soup for 1 hour on High.

Nutritional info per serve: 99 calories, 13.5g protein, 5.4g carbohydrates, 2.3g fat, 0.4g fiber, 40mg cholesterol, 1084mg sodium, 259mg potassium.

Cream of Chicken Soup

Yield: 5 servings | **Prep time:** 10 minutes | **Cook time:** 6 hours

Ingredients:

- 1-pound chicken fillet
- 5 cups chicken stock
- 1 cup heavy cream
- 1 tablespoon smoked paprika

- ½ cup Cheddar cheese, shredded
- ½ cup cauliflower, chopped
- 1 teaspoon ground black pepper

Method:

1. Put the chicken in the slow cooker.
2. Add chicken stock, heavy cream, smoked paprika, cauliflower, and ground black pepper.
3. Close the lid and cook the mixture for 5 hours on High.
4. After this, remove the chicken from the slow cooker.
5. Blend the remaining slow cooker mixture until smooth.
6. Then return the shredded chicken to the slow cooker.
7. Add Cheddar cheese and cook the soup on High for 1 hour.

Nutritional info per serve: 318 calories, 30.7g protein, 3.1g carbohydrates, 20.1g fat, 0.9g fiber, 125mg cholesterol, 925mg sodium, 332mg potassium.

Meat Spinach Stew

Prep time: 20 minutes | **Cook time:** 30 minutes | **Yield:** 4 servings

Ingredients:
- 2 cups spinach, chopped
- 1-pound beef sirloin, chopped
- 1 teaspoon allspices
- 3 cups chicken broth
- 1 cup of coconut milk
- 1 teaspoon coconut aminos

Method:
1. Put all ingredients in the slow cooker.
2. Close and seal the lid.
3. After this, set the manual mode (high pressure) and cook the stew for 30 minutes.
4. When the cooking time is finished, allow the natural pressure release for 10 minutes.
5. Stir the stew gently before serving.

Nutritional info per serve: 383 calories, 39.9g protein, 5.1g carbohydrates, 22.5g fat, 1.8g fiber, 101mg cholesterol, 670mg sodium, 585mg potassium.

Light Zucchini Soup

Yield: 4 servings | **Prep time:** 15 minutes | **Cook time:** 30 minutes

Ingredients:
- 1 large zucchini
- 1 white onion, diced
- 4 cups beef broth
- 1 teaspoon dried thyme
- ½ teaspoon dried rosemary

Method:
1. Pour the beef broth into the slow cooker.
2. Add onion, dried thyme, and dried rosemary.
3. After this, make the spirals from the zucchini with the help of the spiralizer and transfer them to the slow cooker.
4. Close the lid and cook the sou on High for 30 minutes.

Nutritional info per serve: 64 calories, 6.2g protein, 6.5g carbohydrates, 1.6g fat, 1.6g fiber, 0mg cholesterol, 773mg sodium, 462mg potassium.

Tomatillos Fish Stew

Prep time: 15 minutes | **Cook time:** 12 minutes | **Yield:** 2 servings

Ingredients:
- 2 tomatillos, chopped
- 10 oz salmon fillet, chopped
- 1 teaspoon ground
- paprika
- ½ teaspoon ground turmeric
- 1 cup coconut milk

Method:
1. Put all ingredients in the slow cooker.
2. Close and seal the lid.
3. Cook the fish stew on manual mode (high pressure) for 12 minutes.
4. Then allow the natural pressure release for 10 minutes.

Nutritional info per serve: 479 calories, 30.8g protein, 9.6g carbohydrates, 37.6g fat, 3.8g fiber, 63mg cholesterol, 81mg sodium, 990mg potassium.

Bok Choy Soup

Prep time: 5 minutes | **Cook time:** 2 minutes | **Yield:** 1 serving

Ingredients:
- 1 bok choy stalk, chopped
- ¼ teaspoon nutritional yeast
- ½ teaspoon onion
- powder
- ¼ teaspoon chili flakes
- 1 cup chicken broth

Method:
1. Put all ingredients from the list above in the slow cooker.
2. Close and seal the lid and cook the soup on manual (high pressure) for 2 minutes.
3. Make a quick pressure release.

Nutritional info per serve: 55 calories, 6.4g protein, 3.8g carbohydrates, 1.6g fat, 1g fiber, 0mg cholesterol, 810mg sodium, 415mg potassium.

Garlic Soup

Yield: 4 servings | **Prep time:** 10 minutes | **Cook time:** 8 hours

Ingredients:
- 1 teaspoon minced garlic
- 1 cup celery stalk, chopped
- 1 cup daikon, chopped
- 5 cups of water
- 1 teaspoon ground paprika
- 1 tablespoon keto tomato paste

Method:
1. Put all ingredients in the slow cooker and carefully stir until tomato paste is dissolved.
2. Then close the lid and cook the soup on low for 8 hours.

Nutritional info per serve: 13 calories, 0.7g protein, 2.7g carbohydrates, 0.1g fat, 1.1g fiber, 0mg cholesterol, 34mg sodium, 154mg potassium.

Mexican Style Soup

Yield: 6 servings | **Prep time:** 10 minutes | **Cook time:** 5 hours

Ingredients:
- 1-pound chicken fillet, cut into strips
- 2 tablespoons keto enchilada sauce
- 6 cups chicken stock
- 1 cup cauliflower, chopped
- 2 tomatoes, chopped
- 1 teaspoon garlic powder
- ¼ cup fresh cilantro, chopped

Method:
1. Put all ingredients in the slow cooker and close the lid.
2. Cook the soup on high for 5 hours.
3. When the time is finished, open the lid and carefully mix the soup with the help of the ladle.

Nutritional info per serve: 168 calories, 23.3g protein, 3.8g carbohydrates, 6.3g fat, 1.1g fiber, 67mg cholesterol, 872mg sodium, 366mg potassium.

Paprika Noodle Soup

Yield: 4 servings | **Prep time:** 10 minutes | **Cook time:** 1 hour

Ingredients:
- 1 cup zucchini, noodles
- 3 cups chicken stock
- 1 teaspoon butter
- 1 teaspoon ground paprika
- 2 tablespoons fresh parsley, chopped

Method:
1. Put zucchini noodles in the slow cooker.
2. Add chicken stock, butter, ground paprika, and salt.
3. Close the lid and cook the soup on High for 1 hour.
4. Then open the lid, add parsley, and stir the soup.

Nutritional info per serve: 47 calories, 1.6g protein, 6.3g carbohydrates, 1.9g fat, 0.5g fiber, 9mg cholesterol, 873mg sodium, 42mg potassium.

Butternut Squash Soup

Yield: 5 servings | **Prep time:** 15 minutes | **Cook time:** 7 hours

Ingredients:
- 2 cups butternut squash, chopped
- 3 cups chicken stock
- 1 cup heavy cream
- 1 teaspoon ground cardamom
- 1 teaspoon ground cinnamon

Method:
1. Put the butternut squash in the slow cooker.
2. Sprinkle it with ground cardamom and ground cinnamon.
3. Then add chicken stock.
4. Close the lid and cook the soup on High for 5 hours.
5. Then blend the soup until smooth with the help of the immersion blender and add heavy cream.
6. Cook the soup on high for 2 hours more.

Nutritional info per serve: 125 calories, 1.7g protein, 10.5g carbohydrates, 9.3g fat, 2g fiber, 33mg cholesterol, 485mg sodium, 301mg potassium.

Rutabaga Soup

Yield: 6 servings | **Prep time:** 10 minutes | **Cook time:** 4 hours

Ingredients:
- 2 cups rutabaga, peeled, chopped
- 1 cup cauliflower, chopped
- 1 teaspoon chili powder
- 1 teaspoon Italian seasonings
- ¼ cup cherry tomatoes
- 4 cups chicken stock

Method:
1. Put all ingredients in the slow cooker.
2. Close the lid and cook the soup on High for 4 hours.

Nutritional info per serve: 33 calories, 1.5g protein, 5.8g carbohydrates, 0.8g fat, 1.8g fiber, 1mg cholesterol, 528mg sodium, 244mg potassium.

Shrimp Chowder

Yield: 4 servings | **Prep time:** 5 minutes | **Cook time:** 1 hour

Ingredients:
- 1-pound shrimps
- ½ cup fennel bulb, chopped
- 1 bay leaf
- ½ teaspoon
- peppercorn
- 1 cup of coconut milk
- 3 cups of water
- 1 teaspoon ground coriander

Method:
1. Put all ingredients in the slow cooker.
2. Close the lid and cook the chowder on High for 1 hour.

Nutritional info per serve: 277 calories, 27.4g protein, 6.1g carbohydrates, 16.3g fat, 1.8g fiber, 239mg cholesterol, 297mg sodium, 401mg potassium.

Taco Soup

Yield: 3 servings | **Prep time:** 10 minutes | **Cook time:** 8 hours

Ingredients:

- 1 cup ground chicken
- 3 cup chicken stock
- 1 tomato, chopped
- 1 jalapeno pepper, sliced
- 1 tablespoon taco seasoning
- ¼ cup black olives, sliced
- 3 keto tortillas, chopped

Method:

1. Put the ground chicken in the slow cooker.
2. Add chicken stock, tomato, jalapeno pepper, taco seasoning, and black olives.
3. Close the lid and cook the soup on low for 8 hours.
4. When the soup is cooked, ladle it in the bowls and top with chopped tortillas.

Nutritional info per serve: 276 calories, 26.5g protein, 12.5g carbohydrates, 13.3g fat, 4.7g fiber, 42mg cholesterol, 1353mg sodium, 188mg potassium.

Spiced Lasagna Soup

Yield: 6 servings | **Prep time:** 20 minutes | **Cook time:** 6 hours

Ingredients:

- 2 sheets of keto lasagna noodles, crushed
- 1 oz Parmesan, grated
- 1 teaspoon ground turmeric
- 1 yellow onion, diced
- 2 cups ground beef
- 6 cups beef broth
- 2 tomatoes, chopped
- 1 tablespoon dried basil

Method:

1. Roast the ground beef in the hot skillet for 4 minutes. Stir it constantly and transfer it to the slow cooker.
2. Add turmeric, onion, tomatoes, basil, and beef broth.
3. Stir the soup, add keto lasagna noodles, and close the lid.
4. Cook the soup on High for 6 hours.
5. Top the cooked soup with Parmesan.

Nutritional info per serve: 101 calories, 11g protein, 4.6g carbohydrates, 4.2g fat, 1g fiber, 16mg cholesterol, 822mg sodium, 402mg potassium.

Cheese and Rutabaga Soup

Yield: 6 servings | **Prep time:** 15 minutes | **Cook time:** 7 hours

Ingredients:

- 1 cup onion, diced
- 5 cups of water
- 2 cups rutabaga, peeled, chopped
- 1 teaspoon dried
- parsley
- 1 garlic clove
- 1 oz Parmesan, grated
- 1 cup heavy cream

Method:

1. Put the onion in the slow cooker.
2. Add water, rutabaga, parsley, peeled garlic clove, and heavy cream.
3. Close the lid and cook the soup on low for 7 hours.
4. When the time is finished, mash the soup gently with the help of the potato mash.
5. Add Parmesan and stir the soup.

Nutritional info per serve: 131 calories, 3.1g protein, 11.5g carbohydrates, 8.5g fat, 1.9g fiber, 31mg cholesterol, 68mg sodium, 281mg potassium.

White Mushroom Soup

Yield: 6 servings | **Prep time:** 15 minutes | **Cook time:** 8 hours

Ingredients:

- 9 oz white mushrooms, chopped
- 6 chicken stock
- 1 teaspoon dried cilantro
- ½ teaspoon ground
- black pepper
- 1 teaspoon butter
- 1 cup cauliflower, chopped

Method:

1. Melt butter in the skillet.
2. Add white mushrooms and roast them for 5 minutes on high heat. Stir the mushrooms constantly.
3. Transfer them to the slow cooker.
4. Add chicken stock, cilantro, ground black pepper, and cauliflower.
5. Close the lid.
6. Cook the soup on low for 8 hours.

Nutritional info per serve: 44 calories, 2.5g protein, 6.7g carbohydrates, 1.4g fat, 1.2g fiber, 2mg cholesterol, 776mg sodium, 271mg potassium.

Lobster Soup

Yield: 4 servings | **Prep time:** 10 minutes | **Cook time:** 2 hours

Ingredients:

- 4 cups of water
- 1-pound lobster tail, chopped
- ½ cup fresh cilantro, chopped
- 1 cup coconut cream
- 1 teaspoon ground coriander
- 1 garlic clove, diced

Method:

1. Pour water and coconut cream into the slow cooker.
2. Add a lobster tail, cilantro, and ground coriander.
3. Then add the garlic clove and close the lid.
4. Cook the lobster soup on High for 2 hours.

Nutritional info per serve: 241 calories, 23g protein, 3.6g carbohydrates, 15.2g fat, 1.4g fiber, 165mg cholesterol, 568mg sodium, 435mg potassium.

Light Minestrone Soup

Yield: 4 servings | **Prep time:** 7 minutes | **Cook time:** 3 hours

Ingredients:

- 1 cup bean sprouts
- 1 small zucchini, chopped
- 5 cups chicken stock
- 1 teaspoon curry powder
- 2 tablespoons keto tomato paste
- ½ cup ground pork

Method:

1. Put all ingredients in the slow cooker bowl.
2. Close the lid and cook the soup on High for 3 hours.

Nutritional info per serve: 195 calories, 14.6g protein, 13.3g carbohydrates, 9.8g fat, 3.9g fiber, 37mg cholesterol, 999mg sodium, 493mg potassium.

Squash Soup

Yield: 6 servings | **Prep time:** 15 minutes | **Cook time:** 4 hours

Ingredients:

- 1 cup rutabaga, chopped
- 1 cup zucchini
- 1 teaspoon ground turmeric
- 1 teaspoon curry powder
- 1 cup heavy cream
- 4 cups of water

Method:

1. Put rutabaga and zucchini slow cooker.
2. Add ground turmeric and water.
3. Then mix the curry powder and heavy cream and pour the liquid over the vegetables.
4. Close the lid and cook the soup for 4 hours on High.
5. Blend the soup with the help of the immersion blender if desired.

Nutritional info per serve: 109 calories, 1.3g protein, 9.7g carbohydrates, 7.6g fat, 1.8g fiber, 27mg cholesterol, 37mg sodium, 248mg potassium.

Keto Broccoli Soup

Yield: 5 servings | **Prep time:** 10 minutes | **Cook time:** 8 hours

Ingredients:

- ¼ cup keto
- 5 cups chicken stock
- 4 oz pork tenderloin, chopped
- 1 tablespoon dried
- cilantro
- 1 tablespoon keto tomato paste
- ½ cup heavy cream

Method:

1. Put pork tenderloin in the slow cooker.
2. Add broccoli rice, chicken stock, tomato paste, and heavy cream.
3. Carefully stir the soup mixture and close the lid.
4. Cook it on Low for 8 hours.

Nutritional info per serve: 126 calories, 8.3g protein, 10.1g carbohydrates, 6g fat, 2.2g fiber, 33mg cholesterol, 797mg sodium, 249mg potassium.

Tender Mushroom Stew

Yield: 6 servings | **Prep time:** 10 minutes | **Cook time:** 8 hours

Ingredients:

- 1-pound cremini mushrooms, chopped
- 1 yellow onion, diced
- 2 teaspoons dried basil
- ½ cup greek yogurt
- ½ cup rutabaga, chopped
- 5 cups beef broth

Method:

1. Put all ingredients in the slow cooker.
2. Close the lid and cook the stew on Low for 8 hours.

Nutritional info per serve: 77 calories, 8g protein, 7.2g carbohydrates, 1.6g fat, 1.1g fiber, 1mg cholesterol, 649mg sodium, 601mg potassium

Bean Sprouts Chowder

Yield: 6 servings | **Prep time:** 10 minutes | **Cook time:** 8 hours

Ingredients:

- 1-pound chicken breast, skinless, boneless, chopped
- 6 cups of water
- 1 cup bean sprouts
- ¼ cup Greek Yogurt
- 1 tablespoon dried basil
- 1 teaspoon ground black pepper

Method:

1. Mix chicken breast, ground black pepper, and dried basil.
2. Transfer the ingredients to the slow cooker.
3. Add water, bean sprouts, yogurt, and close the lid.
4. Cook the chowder on Low for 8 hours.

Nutritional info per serve: 113 calories, 18.2g protein, 4.1g carbohydrates, 2.2g fat, 1.3g fiber, 49mg cholesterol, 244mg sodium, 359mg potassium.

German Style Soup

Yield: 6 servings | **Prep time:** 10 minutes | **Cook time:** 8.5 hours

Ingredients:

- 1-pound beef loin, chopped
- 6 cups of water
- 1 cup sauerkraut
- 1 onion, diced
- 1 teaspoon cayenne pepper
- ½ cup Greek yogurt

Method:

1. Put beef and onion in the slow cooker.
2. Add yogurt, water, and cayenne pepper.
3. Cook the mixture on low for 8 hours.
4. When the beef is cooked, add sauerkraut and stir the soup carefully.
5. Cook the soup on high for 30 minutes.

Nutritional info per serve: 137 calories, 16.1g protein, 4.3g carbohydrates, 5.8g fat, 1.1g fiber, 41mg cholesterol, 503mg sodium, 93mg potassium.

Chorizo Soup

Yield: 6 servings | **Prep time:** 10 minutes | **Cook time:** 5 hours

Ingredients:

- 9 oz keto chorizo, chopped
- 7 cups of water
- 1 cup cauliflower, chopped
- 1 teaspoon minced garlic, chopped
- 1 zucchini, chopped
- ½ cup spinach, chopped

Method:

1. Put the chorizo in the skillet and roast it for 2 minutes per side on high heat.
2. Then transfer the chorizo to the slow cooker.
3. Add water, cauliflower, minced garlic, zucchini, spinach, and salt.
4. Close the lid and cook the soup on high for 5 hours.
5. Then cool the soup to room temperature.

Nutritional info per serve: 210 calories, 11g protein, 4.3g carbohydrates, 16.4g fat, 0.7g fiber, 37mg cholesterol, 927mg sodium, 326mg potassium.

Bamboo Shoots Soup

Yield: 4 servings | **Prep time:** 10 minutes | **Cook time:** 3.5 hours

Ingredients:

- 1 tablespoon chives, chopped
- 1 teaspoon ground ginger
- 8 oz salmon fillet, chopped
- 5 oz bamboo shoots, canned, chopped
- 1 teaspoon keto hot sauce
- 5 cups of water

Method:

1. Put bamboo shoots in the slow cooker.
2. Add ground ginger, salmon, and water.
3. Close the lid and cook the soup for 3 hours on high.
4. Then add hot sauce and chives. Stir the soup carefully and cook for 30 minutes on high.

Nutritional info per serve: 120 calories, 14.6g protein, 7.9g carbohydrates, 3.8g fat, 3.1g fiber, 25mg cholesterol, 70mg sodium, 612mg potassium

Greens and Coconut Soup

Prep time: 10 minutes | **Cook time:** 4 hours | **Yield:** 6 servings

Ingredients:

- ½ cup fresh spinach, chopped
- 1 cup coconut cream
- 4 cups of water
- 1 cup leek, chopped
- 1-pound chicken breast, skinless, boneless, chopped

Method:

1. Put all ingredients in the slow cooker and close the lid.
2. Cook the soup on High for 4 hours.

Nutritional info per serve: 188 calories, 17.2g protein, 4.4g carbohydrates, 11.5g fat, 1.2g fiber, 48mg cholesterol, 54mg sodium, 427mg potassium.

Celery Soup with Ham

Yield: 8 servings | **Prep time:** 10 minutes | **Cook time:** 5 hours

Ingredients:
- 8 oz ham, chopped
- 8 cups chicken stock
- 1 teaspoon white pepper
- ½ teaspoon cayenne pepper
- 2 cups celery stalk, chopped

Method:
1. Put all ingredients in the slow cooker and gently stir.
2. Close the lid and cook the soup on High for 5 hours.
3. When the soup is cooked, cool it to room temperature and ladle it into the bowls.

Nutritional info per serve: 69 calories, 5.9g protein, 4.6g carbohydrates, 3.2g fat, 1.1g fiber, 16mg cholesterol, 1155mg sodium, 193mg potassium.

Clam Soup

Yield: 2 servings | **Prep time:** 10 minutes | **Cook time:** 1.5 hours

Ingredients:
- ¼ teaspoon ground black pepper
- ¼ teaspoon chili flakes
- 3 cups fish stock
- 8 oz clams, canned
- 1 oz scallions, chopped
- 2 tablespoons Greek yogurt
- ½ teaspoon dried thyme

Method:
1. Pour the fish stock into the slow cooker.
2. Add canned clams, chili flakes, ground black pepper, scallions, and dried thyme.
3. Add Greek yogurt and dried thyme.
4. Cook the soup on High for 1.5 hours.

Nutritional info per serve: 120 calories, 8.9g protein, 13.8g carbohydrates, 3.1g fat, 1g fiber, 4mg cholesterol, 958mg sodium, 649mg potassium.

Turmeric Squash Soup

Yield: 6 servings | **Prep time:** 10 minutes | **Cook time:** 9 hours

Ingredients:
- 3 chicken thighs, skinless, boneless, chopped
- 3 cups butternut squash, chopped
- 1 teaspoon ground turmeric
- 1 yellow onion, sliced
- 1 oz green chilies, chopped
- 6 cups of water

Method:
1. Put chicken thighs in the bottom of the slow cooker and top them with green chilies.
2. Then add the ground turmeric, butternut squash, and water.
3. Add sliced onion and close the lid.
4. Cook the soup on low for 9 Hours.

Nutritional info per serve: 194 calories, 22.6g protein, 13.4g carbohydrates, 5.8g fat, 3.2g fiber, 65mg cholesterol, 78mg sodium, 551mg potassium.

Ground Pork Soup

Yield: 4 servings | **Prep time:** 10 minutes | **Cook time:** 5.5 hour

Ingredients:
- 1 cup ground pork
- 4 cups of water
- 1 tablespoon dried cilantro
- 1 cup Greek yogurt

Method:
1. Put all ingredients in the slow cooker and close the lid.
2. Cook the meal on high for 5.5 hours.

Nutritional info per serve: 101 calories, 10.5g protein, 2g carbohydrates, 5.4g fat, 0g fiber, 23mg cholesterol, 39mg sodium, 151mg potassium.

Lamb Stew

Yield: 5 servings | **Prep time:** 15 minutes | **Cook time:** 5 hours

Ingredients:
- 1-pound lamb meat, cubed
- 1 red onion, sliced
- 1 teaspoon cayenne pepper
- 1 teaspoon dried rosemary
- ½ teaspoon dried thyme
- 1 cup cauliflower, chopped
- 4 cups of water

Method:
1. Sprinkle the lamb meat with cayenne pepper, dried rosemary, and dried thyme.
2. Transfer the meat to the slow cooker.
3. Add water, onion, and cauliflower.
4. Close the lid and cook the stew on high for 5 hours.

Nutritional info per serve: 216 calories, 17.7g protein, 7.2g carbohydrates, 12.2g fat, 1.4g fiber, 64mg cholesterol, 73mg sodium, 166mg potassium.

Keto Tomato Stew

Yield: 4 servings | **Prep time:** 10 minutes | **Cook time:** 7 hours

Ingredients:
- 2 tablespoons keto tomato paste
- 5 cups of water
- 1 yellow onion, chopped
- ½ cup fresh parsley, chopped
- 1 teaspoon ground black pepper
- 2 zucchinis, chopped

Method:
1. Mix tomato paste with water and pour in the slow cooker.
2. Add onion, parsley, zucchinis, and ground black pepper.
3. Close the lid and cook the stew on Low for 7 hours.

Nutritional info per serve: 38 calories, 2g protein, 8.4g carbohydrates, 0.3g fat, 2.6g fiber, 0mg cholesterol, 29mg sodium, 431mg potassium.

Hot Soup

Yield: 4 servings | **Prep time:** 15 minutes | **Cook time:** 24.5 hours

Ingredients:
- ½ cup rutabaga, peeled, diced
- 1 cup cauliflower rice
- 5 cups chicken stock
- 1 onion, diced
- 1 teaspoon chili powder
- 1 teaspoon cayenne pepper
- 1 teaspoon olive oil
- 1 tablespoon keto hot sauce

Method:
1. Roast the onion in olive oil until light brown and transfer to the slow cooker.
2. Add cauliflower rice, chicken stock, rutabaga, chili powder, cayenne pepper, and hot sauce.
3. Carefully stir the soup mixture.
4. Close the lid and cook the soup on High for 4.5 hours.

Nutritional info per serve: 49 calories, 2g protein, 6.9g carbohydrates, 2.2g fat, 2g fiber, 0mg cholesterol, 973mg sodium, 215mg potassium.

Coconut Cod Stew

Yield: 6 servings | **Prep time:** 15 minutes | **Cook time:** 6.5 hours

Ingredients:
- 1-pound cod fillet, chopped
- 2 oz scallions, roughly chopped
- 1 cup coconut cream
- 1 teaspoon curry powder
- 1 teaspoon garlic, diced

Method:
1. Mix curry powder with coconut cream and garlic.
2. Add scallions and gently stir the liquid.
3. After this, pour it into the slow cooker and add cod fillet.
4. Stir the stew mixture gently and close the lid.
5. Cook the stew on low for 6.5 hours.

Nutritional info per serve: 158 calories, 14.7g protein, 3.3g carbohydrates, 10.3g fat, 1.3g fiber, 37mg cholesterol, 55mg sodium, 138mg potassium.

Celery Stew

Yield: 4 servings | **Prep time:** 15 minutes | **Cook time:** 6 hours

Ingredients:
- 3 cups of water
- 1-pound beef stew meat, cubed
- 2 cups celery, chopped
- ½ cup cremini mushrooms, sliced
- 2 tablespoons Greek yogurt
- 1 teaspoon smoked paprika
- 1 teaspoon cayenne pepper
- 1 tablespoon olive oil

Method:
1. Mix beef stew meat with cayenne pepper and put in the hot skillet.
2. Add olive oil and roast the meat for 1 minute per side on high heat.
3. Transfer the meat to the slow cooker.
4. Add celery, cremini mushrooms, Greek yogurt, smoked paprika, and water.
5. Close the lid and cook the stew on high for 6 hours.

Nutritional info per serve: 267 calories, 35.3g protein, 2.7g carbohydrates, 12g fat, 1.2g fiber, 104g cholesterol, 124mg sodium, 660mg potassium.

Bell Pepper Stew

Yield: 3 servings | **Prep time:** 10 minutes | **Cook time:** 5 hours

Ingredients:
- ½ cup bell pepper, chopped
- ¼ cup onion, chopped
- 1 cup butternut squash, chopped
- 1 teaspoon cayenne pepper
- 5 cups of water
- 2 tablespoons cream cheese

Method:

1. Mix water with cream cheese and pour the liquid into the slow cooker.
2. Add cayenne pepper, butternut squash, and onion.
3. Then add bell pepper.
4. Close the lid and cook the stew on high for 5 hours.

Nutritional info per serve: 74 calories, 3.4g protein, 7.9g carbohydrates, 3.6g fat, 2.4g fiber, 7mg cholesterol, 109mg sodium, 218mg potassium.

Italian Style Stew

Yield: 4 servings | **Prep time:** 10 minutes | **Cook time:** 6 hours

Ingredients:

- 2 cups chicken stock
- 1 cup daikon, chopped
- 1 eggplant, chopped
- 1 cup of water
- 1 teaspoon Italian seasonings

Method:

1. Mix chicken stock with daikon and water.
2. Pour the mixture into the slow cooker.
3. Add eggplants and Italian seasonings.
4. Cook the stew on low for 6 hours.

Nutritional info per serve: 40 calories, 1.7g protein, 7.7g carbohydrates, 0.8g fat, 4.3g fiber, 1mg cholesterol, 389mg sodium, 299mg potassium.

Cauli Soup

Prep time: 10 minutes | **Cook time:** 1 hour | **Yield:** 4 servings

Ingredients:

- ½ cup coconut cream
- 1 cup of water
- 2 cups broccoli florets
- ¼ cup spring onions, diced
- ½ teaspoon garlic powder
- 1 cup Cheddar cheese, shredded
- 3 oz bacon, chopped

Method:

1. Mix water and coconut cream and pour it into the slow cooker.
2. Add broccoli florets, spring onion, bacon, and garlic powder. Cook the soup on High for 1 hour.
3. Add cheese and stir the soup until the cheese is dissolved.

Nutritional info per serve: 317 calories, 17g protein, 6.1g carbohydrates, 25.6g fat, 2g fiber, 53mg cholesterol, 689mg sodium, 392mg potassium.

Noodle Soup

Prep time: 10 minutes | **Cook time:** 1.5 hours | **Yield:** 6 servings

Ingredients:

- 2 scallions, diced
- 1 jalapeño pepper, chopped
- 1 tablespoon avocado oil
- 1 teaspoon curry
- powder
- 6 cups chicken stock
- 1-pound chicken breasts, boneless, skinless, and sliced
- 1 zucchini, spiralized

Method:

1. Pour avocado oil into the slow cooker and preheat it on saute mode for 1 minute.
2. Add scallions and cook them for 3 minutes.
3. Then add jalapeno pepper, curry powder, chicken stock, and chicken breast.
4. Saute the mixture for 20 minutes.
5. Then add spiralized zucchini and cook the soup for 1 hour on High.

Nutritional info per serve: 165 calories, 23.1g protein, 2.7g carbohydrates, 6.6g fat, 0.8g fiber, 67mg cholesterol, 833mg sodium, 315mg potassium.

Meatballs Soup

Prep time: 15 minutes | **Cook time:** 2.5 hours | **Yield:** 4 servings

Ingredients:

- 1 teaspoon avocado oil
- 2 spring onions, diced
- 1 cup ground beef
- ½ teaspoon ground
- black pepper
- 4 cups of water
- ½ cup of coconut milk
- 1 tablespoon fresh cilantro, chopped

Method:

1. In the mixing bowl, mix ground beef with ground black pepper. Make the meatballs.
2. Preheat the avocado oil in the slow cooker on saute mode.
3. Put the spring onions inside and roast them for 5 minutes on saute mode.
4. Add water and coconut milk.
5. Add meatballs to the soup.
6. Add cilantro and cook the soup on High for 2 hours.

Nutritional info per serve: 131 calories, 6.6g protein, 2.5g carbohydrates, 11g fat, 1g fiber, 19mg cholesterol, 32mg sodium, 191mg potassium.

Lemongrass Soup

Prep time: 10 minutes | **Cook time:** 3.5 hours | **Yield:** 3 servings

Ingredients:

- 4 cups beef broth
- 1 teaspoon lemongrass
- ½ cup heavy cream
- 1-pound shrimps, peeled
- 1 cup broccoli, chopped
- 1 teaspoon chili powder

Method:

1. Pour beef broth and heavy cream into the slow cooker. Saute the liquid for 15 minutes.
2. Add lemongrass, shrimps, broccoli, and chili powder.
3. Close the lid and cook the soup for 3 hours on High.

Nutritional info per serve: 313 calories, 42.3g protein, 6.7g carbohydrates, 12g fat, 1.1g fiber, 346mg cholesterol, 1413mg sodium, 643mg potassium.

Pepper and Chicken Soup

Prep time: 10 minutes | **Cook time:** 40 minutes | **Yield:** 6 servings

Ingredients:

- 4 cups of water
- 1-pound chicken breast, skinless, boneless, chopped
- 1 cup bell pepper, chopped
- ½ cup celery stalk, chopped
- 1 teaspoon avocado oil
- 1 teaspoon dried basil

Method:

1. Put the chicken in the slow cooker and add water. Cook the chicken on Saute mode for 10 minutes.
2. Then add the bell pepper and avocado oil.
3. Add all remaining ingredients and cook the soup on High for 30 minutes.

Nutritional info per serve: 95 calories, 16.3g protein, 1.8g carbohydrates, 2.1g fat, 0.4g fiber, 48mg cholesterol, 51mg sodium, 343mg potassium.

Clam Soup

Prep time: 10 minutes | **Cook time:** 1-hour | **Yield:** 3 servings

Ingredients:

- 1 cup of organic almond milk
- 1 cup of water
- 6 oz clam, chopped
- 1 teaspoon scallions
- ½ teaspoon ground black pepper
- ¾ teaspoon chili flakes
- 1 cup broccoli florets, chopped

Method:

1. Pour almond milk into the slow cooker.
2. Add water and ground black pepper.
3. Then add chili flakes, salt, and broccoli florets. Add calms.
4. Close the lid and cook the soup on High for 1 hour.

Nutritional info per serve: 223 calories, 3.1g protein, 13g carbohydrates, 19.3g fat, 2.9g fiber, 0mg cholesterol, 230mg sodium, 365mg potassium.

Zucchini Cream Soup

Prep time: 10 minutes | **Cook time:** 1 hour 20 minutes | **Yield:** 4 servings

Ingredients:

- 1 cup ground beef
- 3 cups of water
- 1 tablespoon keto tomato paste
- 1 teaspoon Italian seasonings
- 2 scallions, diced
- 1 tablespoon coconut oil
- 1 cup zucchini, chopped

Method:

1. Put the coconut oil in the slow cooker and melt it on saute mode.
2. Add ground beef and Italian seasonings.
3. Then add diced scallions and saute the mixture for 15 minutes.
4. After this, add keto tomato paste, zucchini, and water and cook the soup on high for 1 hour.
5. Then blend the soup until you get the creamy texture and ladle in the bowls.

Nutritional info per serve: 139 calories, 10.9g protein, 2.5g carbohydrates, 9.5g fat, 0.8g fiber, 34mg cholesterol, 45mg sodium, 290mg potassium.

Turnip Soup

Prep time: 10 minutes | **Cook time:** 2 hours 10 minutes | **Yield:** 4 servings

Ingredients:

- 1 cup of water
- 1 cup of organic almond milk
- 1 cup cremini mushrooms, chopped
- 1 tablespoon coconut oil
- 2 oz turnip, chopped
- 1 teaspoon dried parsley
- ½ teaspoon white pepper
- ¾ teaspoon ground paprika
- 1 oz celery stalk, chopped

Method:

1. Melt the coconut oil in the slow cooker on saute mode.

2. Add cremini mushrooms and turnip and saute the ingredients for 10 minutes.

3. Stir the mixture well and add all remaining ingredients.

4. Close the lid and cook the soup on high for 2 hours.

Nutritional info per serve: 179 calories, 2.1g protein, 5.6g carbohydrates, 17.8g fat, 2g fiber, 0mg cholesterol, 27mg sodium, 299mg potassium.

Lobster Soup

Prep time: 10 minutes | **Cook time:** 6 hours | **Yield:** 4 servings

Ingredients:

- 1 teaspoon garlic powder
- 2 scallions, chopped
- 9 oz lobster meat, chopped
- 1 teaspoon keto tomato paste
- ½ cup celery stalk, chopped
- ½ cup coconut cream
- 1 teaspoon dried lemongrass
- ¼ teaspoon lemon zest

Method:

1. Put all ingredients in the slow cooker and close the lid.

2. Cook the soup on Low for 6 hours.

Nutritional info per serve: 135 calories, 13.3g protein, 3.5g carbohydrates, 7.7g fat, 1.2g fiber, 93mg cholesterol, 327mg sodium, 291mg potassium.

Side Dishes

Tofu Quiche

Prep time: 10 minutes | **Cook time:** 8 minutes | **Yield:** 4 servings

Ingredients:
- 8 oz tofu
- ½ cup mushrooms, chopped, fried
- 1 teaspoon nutritional yeast
- 2 tablespoons almond flour
- 1 teaspoon coconut milk
- 1 teaspoon dried dill
- 1 cup water, for cooking

Method:
1. Chop tofu and mix it up with mushrooms, nutritional yeast, almond flour, coconut milk, and dried dill.
2. Then place the mixture in the baking pan and flatten in the shape of the quiche.
3. Pour water into the slow cooker and insert the steamer rack.
4. Place the quiche on the rack and close the lid.
5. Cook the meal on manual mode (high pressure) for 8 minutes. Then make a quick pressure release.

Nutritional info per serve: 128 calories, 8.4g protein, 4.8g carbohydrates, 9.8g fat, 2.4g fiber, 0mg cholesterol, 14mg sodium, 143mg potassium.

Parm Zucchini Noodles

Prep time: 10 minutes | **Cook time:** 5 minutes | **Yield:** 2 servings

Ingredients:
- 1 large zucchini
- 1 garlic clove, diced
- 1 tablespoon coconut oil
- 3 oz Parmesan, grated
- ½ teaspoon chili flakes

Method:
1. Trim the zucchini and make the spirals from it with the help of the spiralizer.
2. Then toss the coconut oil in the slow cooker and melt it on saute mode.
3. Add garlic and chili flakes and cook the ingredients for 2 minutes.
4. After this, add zucchini spirals and cook them for 2 minutes.
5. Add grated Parmesan and mix up the meal well. Cook it for 1 minute more.

Nutritional info per serve: 223 calories, 15.7g protein, 7.5g carbohydrates, 16.2g fat, 1.8g fiber, 30mg cholesterol, 411mg sodium, 430mg potassium.

Kale Stir Fry

Prep time: 10 minutes | **Cook time:** 3 minutes | **Yield:** 4 servings

Ingredients:
- 8 oz asparagus, chopped
- 2 cups kale, chopped
- 2 bell pepper, chopped
- ½ teaspoon minced ginger
- 1 tablespoon avocado oil
- 1 teaspoon apple cider vinegar
- ½ cup of water

Method:
1. In the slow cooker baking pan, mix up together chopped kale, asparagus, bell pepper, minced ginger, apple cider vinegar, and avocado oil.
2. Then pour water into the slow cooker.
3. Insert the steamer rack and place the mold with a kale mixture on it.
4. Close and seal the lid and cook the kale stir fry for 3 minutes on manual mode (high pressure). Make a quick pressure release.

Nutritional info per serve: 53 calories, 2.9g protein, 10.6g carbohydrates, 0.7g fat, 2.7g fiber, 0mg cholesterol, 18mg sodium, 406mg potassium.

Keto Bread

Prep time: 15 minutes | **Cook time:** 30 minutes | **Yield:** 4 servings

Ingredients:
- 4 eggs, beaten
- 1 teaspoon baking powder
- 1 cup almond flour
- 2 tablespoons chia seeds
- 1/3 cup coconut milk
- 1 teaspoon coconut oil, melted
- 1 cup of water

Method:
1. Put all ingredients except water in the mixing bowl and knead the dough.
2. Then place the dough in the baking pan.
3. Pour water and insert the steamer rack into the slow cooker.
4. Put the pan with dough on the steamer rack and close the lid.
5. Cook the bread on manual mode (high pressure) for 30 minutes.
6. Then make a quick pressure release.
7. Open the lid and let the cooked bread cool to room temperature.
8. Remove it from the pan and slice.

Nutritional info per serve: 194 calories, 8.7g protein, 6.5g carbohydrates, 16g fat, 3.7g fiber, 164mg cholesterol, 71mg sodium, 267mg potassium.

Vegan Pepperoni

Prep time: 20 minutes | **Cook time:** 4 minutes | **Yield:** 6 servings

Ingredients:

- ½ cup nutritional yeast
- 1 teaspoon smoked paprika
- 1 teaspoon garlic powder
- ½ cup coconut flour
- 1 tablespoon coconut oil, melted
- 4 tablespoons water
- 1 cup water, for cooking

Method:

1. Blend nutritional yeast, smoked paprika, garlic powder, coconut flour, melted coconut oil, and 4 tablespoons of water.

2. Then transfer the mixture to the sausage link or foil bag. Make the shape of pepperoni. Secure the ends of the pepperoni.

3. Pour water into the slow cooker.

4. Then place the pepperoni in the water.

5. Close and seal the lid.

6. Cook the meal on manual (high pressure) for 4 minutes.

7. Allow the natural pressure release for 10 minutes.

8. Then cool the cooked pepperoni well and slice it.

Nutritional info per serve: 116 calories, 8.3g protein, 12.7g carbohydrates, 4.7g fat, 7.5g fiber, 0mg cholesterol, 29mg sodium, 333mg potassium.

Tempeh Satay

Prep time: 5 minutes | **Cook time:** 4 minutes | **Yield:** 6 servings

Ingredients:

- 15 oz tempeh
- 1 tablespoon coconut aminos
- ½ teaspoon harissa
- 1 tablespoon coconut oil

Method:

1. Chop the tempeh into cubes.

2. Then put the coconut oil and harissa in the slow cooker and melt it on saute mode.

3. Add chopped tempeh and coconut aminos.

4. Cook the meal on saute mode for 2 minutes – for 1 minute from each side.

Nutritional info per serve: 160 calories, 13.2g protein, 7.3g carbohydrates, 10g fat, 0g fiber, 0mg cholesterol, 14mg sodium, 292mg potassium.

Falafel Salad

Prep time: 20 minutes | **Cook time:** 10 minutes | **Yield:** 4 servings

Ingredients:

- 2 cups lettuce, chopped
- 1 tablespoon olive oil
- 1 teaspoon lemon juice
- ½ teaspoon cayenne pepper
- 1 cup cauliflower,
- shredded
- 1 egg, beaten
- 1/3 cup coconut flour
- 1 teaspoon lemon zest, grated
- 2 tablespoons coconut oil

Method:

1. Make the falafel: mix up grated lemon zest, coconut flour, egg, and cauliflower.

2. Then make the small balls (falafel).

3. Melt the coconut oil in the slow cooker on saute mode and add falafel. Place them in one layer,

4. Cook the falafel balls on saute mode for 3-4 minutes per side or until they are golden brown.

5. Meanwhile, in the salad bowl, mix up lettuce, olive oil, lemon juice, and cayenne pepper. Shake the salad well.

6. Then top it with the cooked falafel.

Nutritional info per serve: 121 calories, 2.2g protein, 3.2g carbohydrates, 11.7g fat, 1.3g fiber, 41mg cholesterol, 27mg sodium, 137mg potassium.

Jicama Mash

Prep time: 10 minutes | **Cook time:** 8 minutes | **Yield:** 4 servings

Ingredients:

- 1-pound jicama, peeled, chopped
- 1 tablespoon coconut oil
- 1 tablespoon chives, chopped
- ½ cup of coconut milk

Method:

1. Put all ingredients from the list above in the slow cooker.

2. Close and seal the lid.

3. Cook the jicama for 8 minutes on manual mode (high pressure) and then make a quick pressure release.

4. Then transfer the mixture to the blender and blend until smooth.

Nutritional info per serve: 142 calories, 1.5g protein, 11.7g carbohydrates, 10.7g fat, 6.2g fiber, 0mg cholesterol, 9mg sodium, 251mg potassium.

Teriyaki Eggplants

Prep time: 10 minutes | **Cook time:** 6 minutes | **Yield:** 6 servings

Ingredients:

- 3 eggplants, trimmed
- 2 tablespoons keto teriyaki
- 2 tablespoons
- avocado oil
- ½ teaspoon ground ginger

Method:

1. Heat avocado oil in saute mode for 2 minutes.
2. Meanwhile, slice the eggplants and sprinkle them with teriyaki, and ground ginger.
3. Arrange the eggplant slices in the slow cooker bowl in one layer and cook them on saute mode for 2 minutes from each side.

Nutritional info per serve: 75 calories, 2.8g protein, 16.5g carbohydrates, 1.1g fat, 9.9g fiber, 0mg cholesterol, 6mg sodium, 644mg potassium.

Cauliflower Tikka Masala

Prep time: 10 minutes | **Cook time:** 3 minutes | **Yield:** 6 servings

Ingredients:

- 1-pound cauliflower, chopped
- 1 teaspoon garam masala
- 1 tablespoon coconut oil
- 1 teaspoon ground turmeric
- 3 oz scallions, chopped
- 1 cup of coconut milk

Method:

1. Put all ingredients in the slow cooker and mix them well.
2. Then close and seal the lid.
3. Cook the tikka masala for 3 minutes on manual mode (high pressure).
4. Then allow the natural pressure release for 5 minutes.
5. Shake the cooked meal well before serving.

Nutritional info per serve: 136 calories, 2.7g protein, 7.5g carbohydrates, 12g fat, 3.2g fiber, 0mg cholesterol, 32mg sodium, 383mg potassium.

Herbed Radish

Prep time: 5 minutes | **Cook time:** 10 minutes | **Yield:** 2 servings

Ingredients:

- 2 cups radish, roughly chopped
- 2 tablespoons butter
- 1 teaspoon Italian
- seasonings
- ¼ teaspoon dried rosemary
- ¼ cup of water

Method:

1. Put all ingredients in the slow cooker and mix them up.
2. Saute the meal for 10 minutes, Stir it with the help of the spatula every 3 minutes.

Nutritional info per serve: 128 calories, 0.9g protein, 4.3g carbohydrates, 12.4g fat, 1.9g fiber, 32mg cholesterol, 129mg sodium, 277mg potassium.

Thyme Cabbage

Prep time: 10 minutes | **Cook time:** 5 minutes | **Yield:** 4 servings

Ingredients:

- 1-pound white cabbage
- 1 teaspoon dried thyme
- 2 tablespoons coconut oil
- 1 cup of water

Method:

1. Cut the white cabbage on medium size petals.
2. Then sprinkle it with dried thyme and coconut oil.
3. Put the cabbage petals in the slow cooker pan.
4. After this, pour water and insert the steamer rack into the slow cooker.
5. Put the pan with cabbage on the rack and close the lid.
6. Cook the meal on manual mode (high pressure) for 5 minutes. Make a quick pressure release.

Nutritional info per serve: 88 calories, 1.5g protein, 6.7g carbohydrates, 6.9g fat, 2.9g fiber, 0mg cholesterol, 22mg sodium, 195mg potassium.

Zucchini Fritters

Prep time: 15 minutes | **Cook time:** 10 minutes | **Yield:** 4 servings

Ingredients:

- 2 large zucchinis, grated
- 1 teaspoon ground flax meal
- 1 daikon, diced
- 1 egg, beaten
- 1 tablespoon coconut oil

Method:

1. In the mixing bowl, mix up grated zucchini, ground flax meal, daikon, and egg.
2. Make the fritters from the zucchini mixture.
3. After this, melt the coconut oil on saute mode.
4. Put the zucchini fritters in the hot oil and cook them for 4 minutes from each side or until they are golden brown.

Nutritional info per serve: 76 calories, 3.7g protein, 6.2g carbohydrates, 5g fat, 2.2g fiber, 41mg cholesterol, 34mg sodium, 467mg potassium.

Spiced Broccoli

Prep time: 10 minutes | **Cook time:** 4 minutes | **Yield:** 4 servings

Ingredients:

- 2 cups broccoli florets
- 1 tablespoon lemon juice
- 1 teaspoon lemon zest, grated
- ½ teaspoon chili powder
- 1 tablespoon ground paprika
- 1 cup of water
- 1 teaspoon olive oil

Method:

1. Pour water into the slow cooker and insert the rack.
2. Put broccoli, lemon juice, lemon zest, chili powder, ground paprika, and olive oil in the baking pan and shake gently.
3. Then place the pan on the rack.
4. Close and seal the lid.
5. Cook the broccoli for 4 minutes on manual mode (high pressure).
6. Then make a quick pressure release.

Nutritional info per serve: 33 calories, 1.6g protein, 4.3g carbohydrates, 1.6g fat, 2g fiber, 0mg cholesterol, 21mg sodium, 198mg potassium.

Cauliflower Gnocchi

Prep time: 10 minutes | **Cook time:** 2 minutes | **Yield:** 4 servings

Ingredients:

- 2 cups cauliflower, boiled
- ½ cup almond flour
- 1 tablespoon avocado oil
- 1 cup of water

Method:

1. Mash the cauliflower until you get puree and mix it up with salt, almond flour, and avocado oil.
2. Then make the log from the cauliflower dough and cut it into small pieces.
3. Pour water into the slow cooker.
4. Add gnocchi. Close and seal the lid.
5. Cook the meal on manual mode (high pressure) for 2 minutes.
6. Then allow the natural pressure release and open the lid.
7. Remove the cooked gnocchi from the water.

Nutritional info per serve: 37 calories, 1.8g protein, 3.6g carbohydrates, 2.2g fat, 1.8g fiber, 0mg cholesterol, 18mg sodium, 163mg potassium.

Chives Mushrooms

Prep time: 10 minutes | **Cook time:** 3 minutes | **Yield:** 2 servings

Ingredients:

- 1 cup cremini mushrooms, sliced
- 2 tablespoons chives, chopped
- 1 tablespoon avocado
- oil
- 1 teaspoon keto ranch seasonings
- 1 cup of water

Method:

1. In the mixing bowl, mix up mushrooms, chives, avocado oil, and keto ranch seasonings.
2. Then pour water and insert the steamer rack in the slow cooker.
3. Put the mushroom mixture in the baking pan and transfer it to the steamer rack.
4. Cook the meal on manual mode (high pressure) for 3 minutes.
5. When the time is finished, make a quick pressure release.

Nutritional info per serve: 20 calories, 1.1g protein, 2g carbohydrates, 1g fat, 2.4g fiber, 0mg cholesterol, 6mg sodium, 193mg potassium.

Broccoli Rice Bowl

Prep time: 10 minutes | **Cook time:** 1 minute | **Yield:** 2 servings

Ingredients:

- 1 ½ cup broccoli, shredded
- ½ teaspoon ground turmeric
- 2 tablespoons plain
- cream cheese
- 1 cup water, for cooking

Method:

1. Pour water and insert the steamer rack into the slow cooker.
2. Put the broccoli shred in the bowl and transfer it to the steamer rack.
3. Close and seal the lid and cook it on manual mode (high pressure) for 1 minute + quick pressure release.
4. Transfer the cooked broccoli to the bowl and add turmeric, and cream cheese.
5. Stir it well.

Nutritional info per serve: 60 calories, 2.7g protein, 5.2g carbohydrates, 3.8g fat, 1.9g fiber, 11mg cholesterol, 52mg sodium, 242mg potassium.

Mashed Turnips

Prep time: 10 minutes | **Cook time:** 5 minutes | **Yield:** 4 servings

Ingredients:

- 2 cups turnips, peeled, chopped
- 3 cups of water
- 1 tablespoon coconut
- milk
- 1 oz tempeh, shredded

Method:

1. Put turnips and water in the slow cooker.
2. Close and seal the lid.
3. Cook the turnip on manual mode (high pressure) for 5 minutes. Make a quick pressure release.
4. Then open the lid and transfer the turnip to the blender.
5. Add tempeh and coconut milk.
6. Blend the meal until it is smooth.
7. Transfer the cooked turnips to the serving bowls.

Nutritional info per serve: 40 calories, 1.9g protein, 4.9g carbohydrates, 1.7g fat, 1.1g fiber, 0mg cholesterol, 47mg sodium, 156mg potassium.

Southern Okra

Prep time: 5 minutes | **Cook time:** 4 minutes | **Yield:** 2 servings

Ingredients:

- ½ teaspoon Erythritol
- 1 teaspoon almond flour
- 1 cup okra, sliced
- 1 teaspoon coconut
- oil
- ½ tomato, chopped
- ½ bell pepper, chopped
- ½ cup of water

Method:

1. Put all ingredients in the slow cooker.
2. Close and seal the lid.
3. Then cook the meal on manual mode (high pressure) for 4 minutes.
4. When the time is finished, make a quick pressure release and transfer the meal to the plates.

Nutritional info per serve: 132 calories, 4.4g protein, 9.6g carbohydrates, 9.5g fat, 3.7g fiber, 0mg cholesterol, 12mg sodium, 243mg potassium.

Scallions&Olives Salad

Prep time: 5 minutes | **Cook time:** 4 minutes | **Yield:** 2 servings

Ingredients:

- 4 oz scallions, sliced
- 1 teaspoon coconut oil
- ½ teaspoon Splenda
- ½ cup olives, sliced
- 1 teaspoon avocado oil
- 1 tablespoon fresh parsley, chopped

Method:

1. Put the sliced scallions and coconut oil in the slow cooker.
2. Saute it for 4 minutes or until the scallions are light brown.
3. Then transfer it to the salad bowl.
4. Add sliced olives, parsley, and avocado oil. Stir the salad.

Nutritional info per serve: 85 calories, 1.4g protein, 7.5g carbohydrates, 6.3g fat, 2.7g fiber, 0mg cholesterol, 303mg sodium, 177mg potassium.

Chia Zoodle Salad

Prep time: 10 minutes | **Cook time:** 3 minutes | **Yield:** 6 servings

Ingredients:

- 2 large zucchinis, trimmed
- 1 teaspoon chia seeds
- ¼ teaspoon chili flakes
- 1 tablespoon coconut
- aminos
- ¼ cup chicken broth
- 1 teaspoon avocado oil
- 1 tablespoon scallions, chopped

Method:

1. Make the noodles from the zucchini using the spiralizer.
2. Then put them in the slow cooker and add chicken broth.
3. Saute the zucchini zoodles for 3 minutes and transfer to the serving bowls.
4. Sprinkle the meal with chia seeds, chili flakes, coconut aminos, avocado oil, and scallions.
5. Gently stir the zoodles.

Nutritional info per serve: 30 calories, 1.8g protein, 4.9g carbohydrates, 0.8g fat, 1.8g fiber, 0mg cholesterol, 46mg sodium, 303mg potassium.

Summer Squash Gratin

Prep time: 15 minutes | **Cook time:** 10 minutes | **Yield:** 4 servings

Ingredients:

- 2 zucchinis, sliced
- ½ cup of coconut milk
- 3 oz tofu, shredded
- 1 teaspoon chili flakes
- ½ teaspoon dried dill
- 1 teaspoon coconut oil
- 1 cup water, for cooking

Method:

1. Grease the gratin mold with coconut oil.
2. Then place the sliced zucchini inside.
3. Add coconut milk, tofu, chili flakes, and dried dill.
4. Cover the gratin with foil and place it on the steamer rack.
5. Pour water into the slow cooker.
6. Then transfer the steamer rack with gratin in the slow cooker and close the lid.
7. Cook the gratin on manual mode (high pressure) for 10 minutes.
8. When the time is finished, allow the natural pressure release for 10 minutes.

Nutritional info per serve: 110 calories, 3.7g protein, 5.4g carbohydrates, 9.4g fat, 2g fiber, 0mg cholesterol, 17mg sodium, 372mg potassium.

Beet Hummus

Prep time: 10 minutes | **Cook time:** 35 minutes | **Yield:** 4 servings

Ingredients:

- 8 oz beets, peeled
- 1 teaspoon tahini paste
- ½ teaspoon harissa
- 1 tablespoon lemon juice
- 2 tablespoons olive oil
- 2 cups of water

Method:

1. Put beets and water in the slow cooker.
2. Cook the vegetables on manual mode (high pressure) for 35 minutes.
3. Then make a quick pressure release and open the lid.
4. Chop the beets and put them in the blender.
5. Add tahini paste, harissa, lemon juice, olive oil, and salt.
6. Blend the mixture until smooth.
7. Cool the hummus.

Nutritional info per serve: 95 calories, 1.2g protein, 6.2g carbohydrates, 7.9g fat, 1.3g fiber, 0mg cholesterol, 57mg sodium, 184mg potassium.

Low Carb Budha Bowl

Prep time: 10 minutes | **Cook time:** 5 minutes | **Yield:** 2 servings

Ingredients:

- ½ cup cauliflower, chopped
- ½ cup mushrooms, chopped
- 4 oz bok choy, chopped
- 1 tablespoon avocado oil
- 1 tablespoon lemon juice
- 1 cup water, for cooking

Method:

1. Pour water and insert the steamer into the slow cooker.
2. Put all vegetables in the steamer; close and seal the lid.
3. Cook the ingredients on steam mode for 5 minutes. Then do the quick pressure release.
4. After this, transfer the cooked vegetables to the serving bowls and sprinkle them with salt, lemon juice, and avocado oil.

Nutritional info per serve: 29 calories, 2.1g protein, 3.7g carbohydrates, 1.1g fat, 1.7g fiber, 0mg cholesterol, 47mg sodium, 306mg potassium.

Portobello Cheese Sandwiches

Prep time: 15 minutes | **Cook time:** 6 minutes | **Yield:** 2 servings

Ingredients:

- 4 Portobello mushrooms caps
- ¼ teaspoon minced garlic
- 1 tablespoon olive oil
- 2 Cheddar cheese slices
- 1 cup water, for cooking

Method:

1. In the shallow bowl mix up garlic and olive oil.
2. Brush the mushrooms with garlic mixture and place them on the trivet.
3. Pour water into the slow cooker. Transfer the trivet with mushroom caps inside.
4. Close and seal the lid and cook the vegetables for 6 minutes on manual mode (high pressure).
5. Then make a quick pressure release and open the lid.
6. Place the cheese slices on 2 mushroom caps and cover them with the remaining mushroom to get the shape of sandwiches.

Nutritional info per serve: 213 calories, 13g protein, 6.5g carbohydrates, 16.3g fat, 2g fiber, 29mg cholesterol, 174mg sodium, 629mg potassium.

Zucchini Hasselback

Prep time: 15 minutes | **Cook time:** 8 minutes |
Yield: 2 servings

Ingredients:
- 2 zucchinis, trimmed
- 2 teaspoons olive oil
- ½ teaspoon white
- pepper
- 1 cup water, for cooking

Method:
1. Cut the zucchinis in the shape of the Hasselback and sprinkle with white pepper, salt, and olive oil.
2. Then place the vegetables on the rack and place it in the slow cooker. Add water.
3. Close and seal the lid and cook the meal on manual mode (high pressure) for 8 minutes.
4. Make a quick pressure release and remove the zucchinis from the slow cooker.

Nutritional info per serve: 73 calories, 2.4g protein, 6.9g carbohydrates, 5g fat, 2.3g fiber, 0mg cholesterol, 20mg sodium, 520mg potassium.

Spiced Cauliflower Head

Prep time: 15 minutes | **Cook time:** 17 minutes |
Yield: 4 servings

Ingredients:
- 13 oz cauliflower head
- 1 tablespoon avocado oil
- 1 tablespoon coconut cream
- 1 teaspoon ground turmeric
- 1 teaspoon ground paprika
- ½ teaspoon ground cumin
- 1 cup of water

Method:
1. Pour water into the slow cooker and insert the steamer rack.
2. In the mixing bowl, mix up avocado oil, coconut cream, ground turmeric, paprika, and ground cumin.
3. Carefully brush the cauliflower head with a coconut cream mixture.
4. Sprinkle the remaining coconut cream mixture over the cauliflower.
5. Transfer the vegetable to the steamer rack.
6. Close and seal the lid.
7. Cook the cauliflower on manual mode (high pressure) for 7 minutes.
8. When the time is finished, allow the natural pressure release for 10 minutes.

Nutritional info per serve: 41 calories, 2.1g protein, 6.1g carbohydrates, 1.6g fat, 2.9g fiber, 0mg cholesterol, 31mg sodium, 332mg potassium.

Turnip Roast

Prep time: 10 minutes | **Cook time:** 10 minutes |
Yield: 2 servings

Ingredients:
- 2 turnips, peeled, chopped
- ½ teaspoon ground paprika
- 1 tablespoon olive oil
- ¼ teaspoon ground black pepper

Method:
1. Sprinkle the chopped turnip with ground paprika, and ground black pepper.
2. Then heat olive oil in the slow cooker on saute mode and add chopped turnip.
3. Cook the turnip on saute mode for 3 minutes from each side.
4. Then close the lid and saute it for 4 minutes more.

Nutritional info per serve: 97 calories, 1.1g protein, 8.5g carbohydrates, 7.1g fat, 2.3g fiber, 0mg cholesterol, 80mg sodium, 246mg potassium.

Butter Mushrooms

Prep time: 10 minutes | **Cook time:** 15 minutes |
Yield: 4 servings

Ingredients:
- 14 oz mushrooms, chopped
- ½ cup coconut milk
- 3 tablespoons butter
- ½ teaspoon dried thyme

Method:
1. Melt the butter in the slow cooker on saute mode and add chanterelle mushrooms.
2. Add dried thyme and saute the vegetables for 5 minutes.
3. Then stir them well and add coconut milk. Close and seal the lid.
4. Cook the mushrooms on manual mode (high pressure) for 10 minutes.
5. Then do the quick pressure release.

Nutritional info per serve: 147 calories, 1g protein, 2g carbohydrates, 15.8g fat, 0.8g fiber, 23mg cholesterol, 66mg sodium, 105mg potassium.

Portobello Steak

Prep time: 7 minutes | **Cook time:** 10 minutes |
Yield: 2 servings

Ingredients:
- 7 oz Portobello mushroom cap
- 1 teaspoon coconut oil
- ¼ teaspoon meat seasonings
- ¼ cup ricotta cheese

Method:

1. Rub the mushrooms with meat seasonings and put them in the slow cooker.

2. Add coconut oil and cook the vegetables on saute mode for 3 minutes per side.

3. Then add ricotta cheese and cook mushroom steaks for 4 minutes more.

Nutritional info per serve: 88 calories, 6g protein, 6.6g carbohydrates, 4.9g fat, 1.5g fiber, 10mg cholesterol, 45mg sodium, 519mg potassium.

Dessert

Butter Truffles

Prep time: 10 minutes | **Cook time:** 5 minutes | **Yield:** 10 servings

Ingredients:

- 3 oz dark chocolate, chopped
- 2 tablespoons butter
- ⅔ cup coconut cream
- 2 tablespoons Erythritol
- ¼ teaspoon vanilla extract
- 1 teaspoon of cocoa powder

Method:

1. Put the chocolate and butter in the slow cooker.
2. Melt the ingredients on saute mode. Stir them from time to time.
3. Add coconut cream, Erythritol, and vanilla extract. Stir until smooth and transfer in the mixing bowl.
4. Then make the small balls (truffles) and coat them in the cocoa powder.
5. Refrigerate the dessert for 10-15 minutes before serving.

Nutritional info per serve: 103 calories, 1.1g protein, 9.1g carbohydrates, 8.7g fat, 0.7g fiber, 8mg cholesterol, 26mg sodium, 79mg potassium.

Pecan Brownies

Prep time: 15 minutes | **Cook time:** 4 hours | **Yield:** 4 servings

Ingredients:

- 3 eggs, beaten
- 2 tablespoons cocoa powder
- 2 teaspoons Erythritol
- ½ cup coconut flour
- 2 pecans, chopped
- ½ cup of coconut milk
- 1 cup water, for cooking

Method:

1. In the mixing bowl, mix eggs with cocoa powder, Erythritol, coconut flour, pecans, and coconut milk.
2. Stir the mixture until smooth and pour it into the brownie mold. Flatten the surface of the brownie batter if needed.
3. Pour water into the slow cooker and insert rack.
4. Place the brownies on the rack and close the lid.
5. Cook the brownies on high for 4 hours.
6. Cool the cooked dessert well.

Nutritional info per serve: 231 calories, 8.1g protein, 14.9g carbohydrates, 17.8g fat, 7.2g fiber, 123mg cholesterol, 81mg sodium, 220mg potassium.

Flaxseeds Doughnuts

Prep time: 20 minutes | **Cook time:** 1 hour | **Yield:** 24 servings

Ingredients:

- ¼ cup erythritol
- ¼ cup flaxseed meal
- ¾ cup coconut flour
- 1 teaspoon baking powder
- 1 teaspoon vanilla
- extract
- 2 eggs, beaten
- 3 tablespoons butter
- ¼ cup heavy cream
- Cooking spray

Method:

1. In the mixing bowl, mix erythritol, flaxseed meal, coconut flour, baking powder, vanilla extract, eggs, butter, and cream.
2. Knead the soft dough and roll up it.
3. Cut the dough into doughnuts with the help of the cutter. Place them in the baking paper squares.
4. Spray the slow cooker mold with cooking spray from inside and put the squares with doughnuts in the slow cooker in one layer.
5. Saute them for 7 minutes per side.

Nutritional info per serve: 47 calories, 1.5g protein, 2.8g carbohydrates, 3.3g fat, 1.8g fiber, 19mg cholesterol, 24mg sodium, 37mg potassium.

Calm Cheesecake

Prep time: 45 minutes | **Cook time:** 4 hours | **Yield:** 8 servings

Ingredients:

- 1 cup cream cheese
- 3 tablespoons Erythritol
- 6 eggs, beaten
- 5 tablespoons water
- 1 cup water, for cooking

Method:

1. Mix cream cheese with eggs, water, and Erythritol. Blend the mixture until smooth.
2. After this, pour 1 cup of water into the slow cooker and insert the slow cooker rack.
3. Transfer the blended cream cheese mixture to the slow cooker mold and flatten gently with the help of the spatula.
4. After this, place the cheesecake on the rack and close the lid.
5. Cook the cheesecake on low for 7 hours.
6. Then cool the cheesecake for 45 minutes in the fridge.

Nutritional info per serve: 148 calories, 6.3g protein, 6.7g carbohydrates, 13.4g fat, 0g fiber, 155mg cholesterol,1321mg sodium, 79mg potassium.

Jelly Bears

Prep time: 20 minutes | **Cook time:** 10 minutes | **Yield:** 7 servings

Ingredients:
- 1 cup of water
- 2 oz strawberries, mashed
- 1 tablespoon gelatin
- 1 teaspoon Erythritol

Method:
1. Put all ingredients in the slow cooker and saute until the mixture is smooth.
2. After this, pour the warm liquid into the silicon molds with the shape of bears and refrigerate until solid.

Nutritional info per serve: 3 calories, 0.1g protein, 0.6g carbohydrates, 0g fat, 0.2g fiber, 0mg cholesterol, 1mg sodium, 13mg potassium.

Pecan Candies

Prep time: 10 minutes | **Cook time:** 3 minutes | **Yield:** 6 servings

Ingredients:
- 5 tablespoons butter, softened
- 4 pecans, chopped
- 1 tablespoon Erythritol
- 1 tablespoon coconut shred

Method:
1. Put butter, pecans, Erythritol, and coconut shred in the slow cooker.
2. Saute the mixture for 3 minutes. Then stir it well until homogenous.
3. Make the small balls from the pecan mixture and refrigerate until solid.

Nutritional info per serve: 155 calories, 1.2g protein, 1.6g carbohydrates, 16.8g fat, 1.1g fiber, 25mg cholesterol, 68mg sodium, 41mg potassium.

Cream Jelly

Prep time: 2 hours | **Cook time:** 5 minutes | **Yield:** 5 servings

Ingredients:
- 2 tablespoons Erythritol
- 1 teaspoon vanilla
- extract
- 2 cups heavy cream
- 2 tablespoons gelatin

Method:
1. Put all ingredients in the slow cooker and cook it for 5 minutes on saute mode.
2. Then stir the mixture well and pour it into the silicone molds.
3. Refrigerate the jelly until solid.

Nutritional info per serve: 168 calories, 1g protein, 3.5g carbohydrates, 17.8g fat, 0g fiber, 66mg cholesterol, 18mg sodium, 37mg potassium.

Cocoa Pie

Prep time: 10 minutes | **Cook time:** 4.5 hours | **Yield:** 5 servings

Ingredients:
- 1 teaspoon baking powder
- 1 teaspoon vanilla extract
- 2 eggs, beaten
- 1 tablespoon of cocoa powder
- 2 tablespoons swerve
- 8 tablespoons coconut cream
- 4 teaspoon coconut flour
- 1 teaspoon avocado oil
- 1 cup of water, for cooking

Method:
1. In the mixing bowl, mix baking powder with vanilla extract, eggs, cocoa powder, swerve, coconut cream, and coconut flour.
2. Stir the mixture until you get a smooth batter.
3. Then brush the slow cooker baking pan with avocado oil and pour the pie batter inside.
4. Pour water into the slow cooker and insert the rack.
5. Place the baking pan with pie on the rack and close the lid.
6. Cook the pie on High for 4.5 hours.

Nutritional info per serve: 99 calories, 3.4g protein, 4.7g carbohydrates, 8.1g fat, 1.7g fiber, 65mg cholesterol, 33mg sodium, 219mg potassium.

Cocoa Muffins

Prep time: 30 minutes | **Cook time:** 12 minutes | **Yield:** 6 servings

Ingredients:
- 6 teaspoons butter
- 1 egg, beaten
- 2 tablespoons Erythritol
- 2 teaspoons cocoa powder
- 1 cup coconut flour
- 1 cup of water, for cooking

Method:
1. Put all ingredients in the mixing bowl and whisk until you get a smooth batter.
2. After this, pour the batter into the muffin molds (fill ½ part of every mold).
3. Pour water into the slow cooker and insert the rack.
4. Place the muffins on the rack and close the lid.
5. Cook the dessert on High for 3.5 hours.

Nutritional info per serve: 126 calories, 3.7g protein, 12.7g carbohydrates, 6.6g fat, 8.2g fiber, 37mg cholesterol, 37mg sodium, 26mg potassium.

Vanilla Mousse

Prep time: 7 minutes | **Cook time:** 7 minutes | **Yield:** 3 servings

Ingredients:
- 2 blackberries, halved
- 1 cup heavy cream
- ½ teaspoon vanilla
- extract
- 2 teaspoon swerve
- 4 tablespoons butter

Method:
1. Put all ingredients in the slow cooker and cook for 5 minutes on saute mode.
2. Then transfer the mixture to the blender and blend for 5 minutes.
3. Transfer the cooked mousse to the serving bowls/glasses.

Nutritional info per serve: 281 calories, 1.1g protein, 3g carbohydrates, 30.2g fat, 0.3g fiber, 96mg cholesterol, 124mg sodium, 43mg potassium.

Pumpkin Pie Spices Cheesecake

Prep time: 10 minutes | **Cook time:** 40 minutes | **Yield:** 8 servings

Ingredients
- 3 tablespoons almond flour
- 1 tablespoon coconut oil, softened
- 3 tablespoons Erythritol
- 1 cup cream cheese
- 1 egg, beaten
- ¼ cup of coconut milk
- 1 teaspoon pumpkin pie spices
- 1 cup water, for cooking

Method
1. In the mixing bowl mix up almond flour, coconut oil, and 1 tablespoon of Erythritol. Knead the dough.
2. Transfer the dough into the cheesecake mold and flatten it to get the pie crust shape. Place it in the freezer for 10 minutes.
3. Meanwhile, put the cream cheese, egg, coconut milk, pumpkin pie spices, and remaining Erythritol in the mixing bowl. Mix the mixture until smooth with the help of the hand mixer.
4. Pour the cream cheese mixture over the frozen pie crust, flatten it well.
5. Pour water and insert the steamer rack in the slow cooker and put the cheesecake on it.
6. Close and seal the lid.
7. Cook it on manual (high pressure) for 30 minutes. Make a quick pressure release.

Nutritional info per serve: 202 calories, 5.3g protein, 9.3g carbohydrates, 19.4g fat, 1.3g fiber, 52mg cholesterol, 99mg sodium, 63mg potassium.

Cheese Pie

Prep time: 40 minutes | **Cook time:** 10 minutes | **Yield:** 12 servings

Ingredients:
- 1 cup coconut, shredded
- 2 tablespoons flax seeds
- ¼ cup of coconut oil
- ½ cup heavy cream
- 1 cup cream cheese
- 3 tablespoons Erythritol
- 1 teaspoon vanilla extract
- 1 tablespoon gelatin

Method:
1. Mix the shredded coconut with flax seeds, coconut oil, heavy cream, cream cheese, Erythritol, and vanilla extract.
2. Whisk the mixture until smooth and add gelatin.
3. Pour the liquid into the slow cooker bowl.
4. Start to preheat the liquid on saute mode until gelatin is melted.
5. Transfer the smooth mixture to the pie mold.
6. Then transfer the pie mold into the baking mold and refrigerate for 40 minutes.

Nutritional info per serve: 155 calories, 2g protein, 5.8g carbohydrates, 15.7g fat, 0.9g fiber, 28mg cholesterol, 61mg sodium, 61mg potassium.

Chocolate Pie

Prep time: 10 minutes | **Cook time:** 4 hours | **Yield:** 8 servings

Ingredients:
- 3 tablespoons coconut oil, softened
- ½ cup coconut milk
- 1 teaspoon baking powder
- 1 cup coconut flour
- 1 oz dark chocolate, chopped
- 1 cup of water, for cooking

Method:
1. Mix coconut oil with baking powder, coconut flour, and coconut cream.
2. Then transfer the mixture to the non-stick slow cooker baking pan. Flatten the surface of the pie with the help of the spatula and top with chopped chocolate.
3. Pour water into the slow cooker and insert rack.
4. Place the pie on the rack and close the lid.
5. Cook the chocolate pie on Low for 4 hours.
6. Cool it well.

Nutritional info per serve: 158 calories, 2.6g protein, 11.2g carbohydrates, 11.7g fat, 5.5g fiber, 1mg cholesterol, 36mg sodium, 116mg potassium.

Blackberries Bars

Prep time: 10 minutes | **Cook time:** 4 hours | **Yield:** 12 servings

Ingredients:

- ½ cup butter
- 2 oz blackberries, chopped
- 2 tablespoons Erythritol
- 2 tablespoons
- coconut flour
- ½ cup coconut, shredded
- 1 cup of water, for cooking

Method:

1. Mix butter with coconut flour and coconut shred and knead the dough.
2. Then put the mixture in the slow cooker baking pan and flatten in the shape of the pie crust.
3. After this, mix blackberries with Erythritol.
4. Top the pie crust with blackberries mixture.
5. Pour water into the slow cooker and insert the rack.
6. Put the baking pan with dessert on the rack and close the lid.
7. Bake the bars on High for 4 hours.
8. Cool them well before serving.

Nutritional info per serve: 87 calories, 0.5g protein, 4.2g carbohydrates, 9g fat, 1.1g fiber, 20mg cholesterol, 58mg sodium, 22mg potassium.

Avocado Mousse

Prep time: 15 minutes | **Cook time:** 5 minutes | **Yield:** 4 servings

Ingredients:

- 1 avocado, peeled, pitted, chopped
- 1/3 cup organic almond milk
- 1 tablespoon Erythritol
- 1 teaspoon vanilla extract

Method:

1. Blend the avocado until smooth.
2. Then add almond milk, Erythritol, and vanilla extract.
3. Pour the mixture into the slow cooker and cook it for 5 minutes on saute mode. Stir the mixture constantly.
4. Carefully stir the cooked mousse last time and transfer it to the serving bowl. Cool it until cold.

Nutritional info per serve: 152 calories, 1.4g protein, 9.3g carbohydrates, 14.6g fat, 3.8g fiber, 0mg cholesterol, 6mg sodium, 298mg potassium.

Coconut Panna Cotta

Prep time: 40 minutes | **Cook time:** 5 minutes | **Yield:** 2 servings

Ingredients:

- 1 cup coconut cream
- 1 teaspoon vanilla extract
- 2 teaspoons Erythritol
- 2 teaspoon coconut shred
- 1 tablespoon gelatin powder

Method:

1. Mix coconut cream with gelatin powder, vanilla extract, and Erythritol.
2. Transfer the mixture to the slow cooker and cook it on saute mode for 5 minutes or until you get a smooth liquid.
3. Pour the cooking liquid into the serving cups.
4. Top every cup with coconut shred and refrigerate for 40 minutes.

Nutritional info per serve: 299 calories, 2.8g protein, 12.6g carbohydrates, 30.3g fat, 3g fiber, 0mg cholesterol, 19mg sodium, 319mg potassium.

Cheesecake Bars

Prep time: 25 minutes | **Cook time:** 2 hours | **Yield:** 8 servings

Ingredients:

- 1 cup cream cheese
- 3 egg, beaten
- ¼ cup of coconut milk
- 3 tablespoons Erythritol
- 1 teaspoon vanilla extract
- ¼ cup coconut flour
- 1 tablespoon butter
- 1 tablespoon flax meal

Method:

1. In the mixing bowl, mix eggs with coconut milk, Erythritol, vanilla extract, coconut flour, butter, and flax meal.
2. Put the mixture in the baking pan and flatten it in the shape of the pie crust. Cover it with foil.
3. Pour water into the slow cooker and insert rack.
4. Place the baking pan on the rack and close the lid.
5. Cook the pie crust for 2 hours on high.
6. Chill the cooked pie crust well and spread it with cream cheese.
7. Cut the meal into bars.

Nutritional info per serve: 175 calories, 5.2g protein, 9.8g carbohydrates, 15.7g fat, 1.9g fiber, 97mg cholesterol, 120mg sodium, 85mg potassium.

Coconut Pudding

Prep time: 20 minutes | **Cook time:** 10 minutes | **Yield:** 2 servings

Ingredients:

- ½ cup coconut cream
- 2 eggs, beaten
- 1 teaspoon coconut flour
- 2 tablespoons Erythritol
- 1 teaspoon vanilla extract

Method:

1. Mix all ingredients and put in the slow cooker bowl.
2. Saute the liquid for 10 minutes, stir it constantly.
3. Transfer the hot liquid to the serving cups and refrigerate for 15-20 minutes.

Nutritional info per serve: 212 calories, 7.1g protein, 9.6g carbohydrates, 18.8g fat, 1.7g fiber, 164mg cholesterol, 73mg sodium, 220mg potassium.

Pecan Pie

Prep time: 20 minutes | **Cook time:** 25 minutes | **Yield:** 4 servings

Ingredients:

- 2 tablespoons butter, softened
- 4 tablespoons almond flour
- 4 pecans, chopped
- 1 tablespoon Erythritol
- 2 tablespoons coconut oil
- 1 tablespoon coconut flour
- 1 cup water, for cooking

Method:

1. Make the pie crust: mix up coconut oil and almond flour in the bowl.
2. Then knead the dough and put it in the baking pan. Flatten the dough in the shape of the pie crust.
3. Then melt Erythritol, butter, and coconut flour.
4. When the mixture is liquid, add chopped pecans.
5. Pour water into the slow cooker and insert the steamer rack.
6. Pour the butter-pecan mixture over the pie crust, flatten it and transfer on the steamer rack.
7. Cook the pecan pie on manual mode (high pressure) for 25 minutes.
8. Allow the natural pressure release for 10 minutes and cool the cooked pie well.

Nutritional info per serve: 257 calories, 3.3g protein, 8.5g carbohydrates, 26.1g fat, 3g fiber, 15mg cholesterol, 43mg sodium, 60mg potassium.

Cream Cheese Mousse

Prep time: 20 minutes | **Cook time:** 10 minutes | **Yield:** 2 servings

Ingredients:

- ½ cup coconut cream
- 3 tablespoons cream cheese
- 1 egg, beaten
- 1 tablespoon Erythritol
- 1 tablespoon coconut shred

Method:

1. Mix coconut cream with coconut shred, Erythritol, and cream cheese. Add egg and mix the mixture until smooth.
2. Transfer the mixture to the slow cooker and cook it on saute mode for 10 minutes. Stir the mixture constantly with the help of the spatula. The mousse is cooked.
3. After this, transfer the mousse to the serving cups and chill it.

Nutritional info per serve: 247 calories, 5.3g protein, 12.4g carbohydrates, 24.2g fat, 1.8g fiber, 98mg cholesterol, 85mg sodium, 205mg potassium.

Coconut Cookies

Prep time: 15 minutes | **Cook time:** 3 hours | **Yield:** 6 servings

Ingredients:

- ½ cup coconut flour
- 2 teaspoons coconut oil
- ¾ teaspoon coconut shred
- 1 teaspoon Erythritol
- 3 tablespoons coconut milk
- 1 cup of water for cooking

Method:

1. In the mixing bowl, mix coconut flour with coconut oil, coconut shred, and Erythritol.
2. Add coconut milk and knead the dough.
3. Then make 6 balls from the dough and press them gently in the shape of the cookies.
4. Pour water into the slow cooker and insert the rack.
5. Put the cookies in the baking mold and place the mold on the rack.
6. Close the lid and cook the dessert on high for 3 hours.

Nutritional info per serve: 78 calories, 2.2g protein, 7.3g carbohydrates, 5.1g fat, 4.2g fiber, 0mg cholesterol, 21mg sodium, 20mg potassium.

Cocoa Fudge

Prep time: 30 minutes | **Cook time:** 10 minutes | **Yield:** 4 servings

Ingredients:

- 4 tablespoons coconut oil
- ¼ cup of coconut milk
- ½ teaspoon vanilla extract
- 2 teaspoons Erythritol
- 3 tablespoons cocoa powder

Method:

1. Put the coconut oil in the slow cooker and mix it with cocoa powder, Erythritol, vanilla extract, and coconut milk. Stir the mixture and cook on saute mode for 10 minutes. Stir it from time to time to avoid burning.

2. Then line the baking mold with baking paper.

3. Pour the hot fudge mixture inside, flatten it and refrigerate for 30 minutes or until it is solid.

4. Cut the fudge into bars.

Nutritional info per serve: 162 calories, 1.1g protein, 5.6g carbohydrates, 17.7g fat, 1.5g fiber, 0mg cholesterol, 3mg sodium, 142mg potassium.

Coconut Cookies

Prep time: 15 minutes | **Cook time:** 4 hours | **Yield:** 6 servings

Ingredients:

- 2 tablespoons coconut shred
- 1 teaspoon vanilla extract
- 3 tablespoons coconut oil
- ½ cup coconut flour
- 1 tablespoon Erythritol
- 1 cup of water, for cooking

Method:

1. Put all ingredients in the mixing bowl and, mix and knead the dough.

2. Make 6 coconut cookies by using a cutter.

3. Pour water into the slow cooker and insert the rack.

4. Place the baking pan on the rack and line it with baking paper.

5. Place the cookies in the baking pan and close the lid.

6. Cook the cookies on High for 4 hours.

Nutritional info per serve: 124 calories, 2g protein, 9.3g carbohydrates, 10.1g fat, 4.3g fiber, 0mg cholesterol, 21mg sodium, 1mg potassium.

Sweet Mousse

Prep time: 10 minutes | **Cook time:** 5 minutes | **Yield:** 5 servings

Ingredients:

- 1 cup heavy cream
- 1 tablespoon Erythritol
- 5 teaspoons cream cheese
- 1 tablespoon coconut flour

Method:

1. Pour the heavy cream into the slow cooker bowl and add coconut flour and Erythritol. Stir the mixture until homogenous.

2. Cook it on saute mode for 5 minutes. Stir it from time to time.

3. Then add cream cheese and whisk the mousse until it is smooth.

4. Transfer it to the serving cups.

Nutritional info per serve: 100 calories, 0.9g protein, 4.8g carbohydrates, 10.2g fat, 0.6g fiber, 37mg cholesterol, 19mg sodium, 22mg potassium.

Daikon Cake

Prep time: 10 minutes | **Cook time:** 45 minutes | **Yield:** 12 servings

Ingredients

- 5 eggs, beaten
- ½ cup coconut milk
- 1 cup almond flour
- 1 daikon, diced
- 1 teaspoon ground cinnamon
- 2 tablespoon Erythritol
- 1 tablespoon coconut oil, melted
- 1 cup water, for cooking

Method

1. In the mixing bowl, mix up eggs, coconut milk, almond flour, ground cinnamon, and Erythritol.

2. When the mixture is smooth, add daikon and coconut oil, and stir it carefully with the help of the spatula.

3. Pour the mixture into the cake pan.

4. Then pour water and insert the steamer rack in the slow cooker.

5. Place the cake in the slow cooker.

6. Close and seal the lid.

7. Cook the cake in manual mode (high pressure) for 45 minutes. Make a quick pressure release.

Nutritional info per serve: 116 calories, 4.6g protein, 5.5g carbohydrates, 9.8g fat, 1.4g fiber, 68mg cholesterol, 31mg sodium, 61mg potassium.

Lemon Pie

Yield: 6 servings | **Prep time:** 15 minutes | **Cook time:** 7 hours

Ingredients:

- ½ lemon, chopped
- 1 cup almond flour
- ¼ cup of coconut oil
- ¼ cup of coconut milk
- 1 teaspoon baking powder
- 3 tablespoons Erythritol
- 1 cup of water, for cooking

Method:

1. Mix almond flour with coconut oil, coconut milk, baking powder, and Erythritol.
2. Transfer the mixture to the non-stick slow cooker baking pan and top with chopped lemon.
3. Pour water into the slow cooker and insert the rack.
4. Place the baking pan with pie on the rack and close the lid.
5. Cook the lemon pie on Low for 7 hours.

Nutritional info per serve: 215 calories, 4.3g protein, 12.9g carbohydrates, 20.3g fat, 2.4g fiber, 0mg cholesterol, 9mg sodium, 117mg potassium.

Avocado Pie

Yield: 6 servings | **Prep time:** 10 minutes | **Cook time:** 6 hours

Ingredients:

- 1 avocado, pitted, peeled, sliced
- 1 cup heavy cream
- 1 ½ cup coconut flour
- 1 teaspoon baking powder
- 3 tablespoons Erythritol
- 1 tablespoon butter
- 1 cup of water, for cooking

Method:

1. Mix coconut flour with heavy cream, baking powder, Erythritol, and butter.
2. Make the smooth mixture and pour it into the slow cooker non-stick baking pan.
3. Top the batter with avocado.
4. Pour water into the slow cooker and insert the rack. Place the avocado pie on the rack and close the lid.
5. Cook the pie on Low for 6 hours.

Nutritional info per serve: 170 calories, 1.6g protein, 13.3g carbohydrates, 16.4g fat, 3.5g fiber, 33mg cholesterol, 32mg sodium, 262mg potassium.

Berries Ice Cream

Yield: 2 servings | **Prep time:** 25 minutes | **Cook time:** 10 minutes

Ingredients:

- 2 raspberries, frozen
- 2 blackberries, frozen
- ½ cup coconut milk

Method:

1. Put the raspberries and blackberries in the food processor and blend until smooth. Then mix the berries with coconut milk.
2. Pour the mixture into the slow cooker and close the lid. Cook the mixture on saute mode for 7 minutes.
3. Then transfer the mixture to the plastic vessel and refrigerate until it is solid.

Nutritional info per serve: 148 calories, 1.6g protein, 5.7g carbohydrates, 14.4g fat, 2.6g fiber, 0mg cholesterol, 9mg sodium, 188mg potassium.

Cocoa Squares

Yield: 9 servings | **Prep time:** 10 minutes | **Cook time:** 7 hours

Ingredients:

- 4 tablespoons butter, softened
- ½ teaspoon baking powder
- 4 tablespoons Erythritol
- 1 teaspoon vanilla extract
- 4 ounces cream cheese
- 6 eggs, beaten
- 3 tablespoons cocoa powder
- 1 cup of water, for cooking

Method:

1. Mix butter with baking powder, Erythritol, vanilla extract, cream cheese, eggs, and cocoa powder.
2. When the mixture is homogenous, transfer it to the slow cooker baking pan.
3. Pour water into the slow cooker and insert the rack.
4. Place the baking pan with dessert mixture on the rack.
5. Close the lid and cook the meal on Low for 7 hours.
6. Cool the dessert well and cut it into squares.

Nutritional info per serve: 137 calories, 5g protein, 8.4g carbohydrates, 12.7g fat, 0.6g fiber, 137mg cholesterol, 115mg sodium, 130mg potassium.

Mint Brownies

Yield: 12 servings | **Prep time:** 10 minutes | **Cook time:** 6 hours

Ingredients:

- 1 cup butter
- 6 eggs, beaten
- 3 tablespoons cocoa powder
- 1 teaspoon vanilla extract
- ½ teaspoon baking powder
- ½ cup coconut cream
- ½ cup coconut flour
- 1 teaspoon dried mint
- 1 cup of water, for cooking

Method:

1. Mix butter with eggs, cocoa powder, vanilla extract, baking powder, coconut cream, coconut flour, and dried mint.
2. When the mixture is smooth, pour it in the slow cooker non-sticky brownie mold.
3. Pour water into the slow cooker and insert the rack.
4. Place the brownie on the rack and close the lid.
5. Cook the meal on Low for 6 hours.
6. Cool the brownie well and cut it into servings.

Nutritional info per serve: 214 calories, 4.1g protein, 5g carbohydrates, 20.6g fat, 2.6g fiber, 123mg cholesterol, 142mg sodium, 117mg potassium.

Berry Muffins

Yield: 8 servings | **Prep time:** 10 minutes | **Cook time:** 4 hours

Ingredients:

- 1/3 cup coconut oil
- 1 teaspoon vanilla extract
- 2 tablespoons Erythritol
- 1 cup coconut flour
- 1 oz raspberries
- 1 egg, beaten
- 1 teaspoon baking powder
- 1 cup of water, for cooking

Method:

1. Put all ingredients except raspberries in the mixing bowl and mix until smooth.
2. Then add raspberries and carefully mix the muffin batter with the help of the spoon.
3. Transfer the mixture to the muffin molds (fill ½ part of every mold.
4. Pour water into the slow cooker and insert the rack.
5. Place the muffins on the rack and close the lid.
6. Cook them on High for 4 hours.

Nutritional info per serve: 150 calories, 2.7g protein, 14.6g carbohydrates, 11.2g fat, 6.2g fiber, 20mg cholesterol, 8mg sodium, 77mg potassium.

Chocolate Bacon Strips

Prep time: 30 minutes | **Cook time:** 10 minutes | **Yield:** 6 servings

Ingredients:

- 6 bacon sliced, cooked
- 2 oz dark chocolate
- 1 tablespoon coconut
- oil
- ¼ teaspoon dried mint

Method:

1. Freeze the bacon slices for 15-20 minutes in the freezer.
2. Meanwhile, put chocolate in the slow cooker. Add coconut oil and dried mint. Cook the ingredients on saute mode for 5-10 minutes or until the chocolate is melted.
3. Then dip every bacon slice in the chocolate mixture and refrigerate for 10-15 minutes.

Nutritional info per serve: 139 calories, 0.7g protein, 5.6g carbohydrates, 7.1g fat, 0.3g fiber, 2mg cholesterol, 269mg sodium, 36mg potassium.

Lime Muffins

Prep time: 10 minutes | **Cook time:** 15 minutes | **Yield:** 6 servings

Ingredients:

- 1 teaspoon lime zest
- 1 tablespoon lemon juice
- 1 teaspoon baking powder
- 1 cup almond flour
- 2 eggs, beaten
- 1 tablespoon swerve
- ¼ cup coconut milk
- 1 cup water, for cooking

Method:

1. In the mixing bowl, mix up lemon juice, baking powder, almond flour, eggs, swerve, and coconut milk.
2. When the muffin batter is smooth, add lime zest and mix it up.
3. Fill the muffin molds with batter.
4. Then pour water and insert the rack in the slow cooker.
5. Place the muffins on the rack. Close and seal the lid.
6. Cook the muffins on manual (high pressure) for 15 minutes.
7. Then allow the natural pressure release.

Nutritional info per serve: 153 calories, 6.1g protein, 5.5g carbohydrates, 13.2g fat, 2.3g fiber, 55mg cholesterol, 23mg sodium, 133mg potassium.

Almond Bars

Yield: 4 servings | **Prep time:** 15 minutes | **Cook time:** 3.5 hours

Ingredients:

- ½ cup almond flour
- 2 oz almonds, chopped
- 3 tablespoons butter
- 1 tablespoon Erythritol
- 1 teaspoon vanilla extract
- ½ teaspoon baking powder
- 1 cup of water, for cooking

Method:

1. Mix almond flour with butter, Erythritol, vanilla extract, and baking powder.
2. Then add almond and knead the dough.
3. Put the dough in the lined with the baking paper slow cooker mold and cut into bars.
4. Pour water into the slow cooker and insert the rack.
5. Place the mold on the rack and close the lid.
6. Cook the almond bars on High for 3.5 hours. Cool the cooked almond bars well.

Nutritional info per serve: 246 calories, 6.1g protein, 10.2g carbohydrates, 22.4g fat, 3.3g fiber, 23mg cholesterol, 67mg sodium, 172mg potassium.

Almond Pie

Prep time: 15 minutes | **Cook time:** 41 minutes | **Yield:** 8 servings

Ingredients

- 1 cup almond flour
- ½ cup of coconut milk
- 1 teaspoon vanilla extract
- 2 tablespoons coconut oil, softened
- 1 tablespoon Truvia
- ¼ cup coconut, shredded
- 1 cup water, for cooking

Method

1. In the mixing bowl, mix up almond flour, coconut milk, vanilla extract, coconut oil, Truvia, and shredded coconut.
2. When the mixture is smooth, transfer it to the baking pan and flatten.
3. Pour water and insert the steamer rack into the slow cooker.
4. Put the baking pan with cake on the rack. Close and seal the lid.
5. Cook the dessert on manual mode (high pressure) for 41 minutes. Allow the natural pressure release for 10 minutes.

Nutritional info per serve: 158 calories, 3.4g protein, 4.9g carbohydrates, 14.5g fat, 2.1g fiber, 0mg cholesterol, 8mg sodium, 49mg potassium.

Coconut Cupcakes

Prep time: 15 minutes | **Cook time:** 10 minutes | **Yield:** 6 servings

Ingredients:

- 4 eggs, beaten
- 4 tablespoons coconut milk
- 4 tablespoons coconut flour
- ½ teaspoon vanilla extract
- 2 tablespoons Erythritol
- 1 teaspoon baking powder
- 1 cup water, for cooking

Method:

1. In the mixing bowl, mix up eggs, coconut milk, coconut flour, vanilla extract, Erythritol, and baking powder.
2. Then pour the batter into the cupcake molds.
3. Pour water and insert the steamer rack into the slow cooker.
4. Place the cupcakes on the rack. Close and seal the lid.
5. Cook the cupcakes for 10 minutes on manual mode (high pressure).
6. Then allow the natural pressure release for 5 minutes.

Nutritional info per serve: 87 calories, 4.6g protein, 9.6g carbohydrates, 5.8g fat, 2.2g fiber, 109mg cholesterol, 43mg sodium, 150mg potassium.

Crème Brule

Prep time: 25 minutes | **Cook time:** 10 minutes | **Yield:** 2 servings

Ingredients:

- 1 cup coconut cream
- 5 egg yolks
- 2 tablespoons
- Erythritol
- 1 cup water, for cooking

Method:

1. Whisk the egg yolks and Erythritol together.
2. Then add coconut cream and stir the mixture carefully.
3. Pour the mixture into ramekins and place them on the steamer rack.
4. Pour water into the slow cooker. Add steamer rack with ramekins.
5. Close and seal the lid.
6. Cook crème Brule for 10 minutes – High pressure. Allow the natural pressure release for 15 minutes.

Nutritional info per serve: 411 calories, 9.5g protein, 12.3g carbohydrates, 39.9g fat, 2.6g fiber, 524mg cholesterol, 38mg sodium, 362mg potassium.

Chocolate Mousse

Prep time: 10 minutes | **Cook time:** 4 minutes | **Yield:** 1 serving

Ingredients:

- 1 egg yolk
- 1 teaspoon Erythritol
- 1 teaspoon of cocoa powder
- 2 tablespoons plain
- coconut milk
- 1 tablespoon cream cheese
- 1 cup water, for cooking

Method:

1. Pour water and insert the steamer rack into the slow cooker.
2. Then whisk the egg yolk with Erythritol.
3. When the mixture turns into lemon color, add coconut milk, cream cheese, and cocoa powder. Whisk the mixture until smooth.
4. Then pour it into the glass jar and place it on the steamer rack.
5. Close and seal the lid.
6. Cook the dessert on manual (high pressure) for 4 minutes. Make a quick pressure release.

Nutritional info per serve: 162 calories, 4.5g protein, 8.5g carbohydrates, 15.4g fat, 1.2g fiber, 221mg cholesterol, 43mg sodium, 155mg potassium.

Raspberry Muffins

Yield: 6 servings | **Prep time:** 15 minutes | **Cook time:** 5 hours

Ingredients:

- 1 teaspoon baking powder
- ¼ cup of Erythritol
- ½ cup raspberries
- 1 egg, beaten
- ½ cup coconut flour
- 1/3 cup heavy cream
- 2 tablespoon butter, melted

Method:

1. Put all ingredients except raspberries in the food processor.
2. Blend the mixture until smooth.
3. Then add raspberries and carefully stir the batter with the help of the spoon.
4. Fill the ½ part of every muffin mold with batter and transfer them to the slow cooker.
5. Close the lid and cook the muffins on Low 5 hours.

Nutritional info per serve: 79 calories, 1.4g protein, 12.5g carbohydrates, 7.3g fat, 1.1g fiber, 47mg cholesterol, 43mg sodium, 115mg potassium.

Anise Hot Chocolate

Prep time: 10 minutes | **Cook time:** 2 minutes | **Yield:** 3 servings

Ingredients:

- 1 tablespoon cocoa powder
- 1 tablespoon Erythritol
- ¼ cup heavy cream
- ½ cup of coconut milk
- ½ teaspoon ground anise

Method:

1. Put all ingredients in the slow cooker bowl. Stir them well until you get a smooth liquid.
2. Close and seal the lid.
3. Cook the hot chocolate on manual (high pressure) for 2 minutes. Then allow the natural pressure release for 5 minutes.

Nutritional info per serve: 131 calories, 1.5g protein, 8.5g carbohydrates, 13.5g fat, 1.4g fiber, 14mg cholesterol, 10mg sodium, 158mg potassium.

Blueberry Muffins

Prep time: 15 minutes | **Cook time:** 14 minutes | **Yield:** 6 servings

Ingredients:

- ¼ cup blueberries
- ¼ teaspoon baking powder
- 1 teaspoon apple cider vinegar
- 4 teaspoons coconut oil, melted
- 2 eggs, beaten
- 1 cup coconut flour
- 2 tablespoons Erythritol
- 1 cup water, for cooking

Method:

1. In the mixing bowl, mix up baking powder, apple cider vinegar, coconut oil, eggs, coconut flour, and Erythritol.
2. When the batter is smooth, add blueberries. Stir well.
3. Put the muffin batter in the muffin molds.
4. After this, pour water and insert the steamer rack into the slow cooker.
5. Then place the muffins on the rack. Close and seal the lid.
6. Cook the muffins on manual mode (high pressure) for 14 minutes.
7. When the time is finished, allow the natural pressure release for 6 minutes.

Nutritional info per serve: 131 calories, 4.6g protein, 19.4g carbohydrates, 6.5g fat, 8.2g fiber, 55mg cholesterol, 21mg sodium, 46mg potassium.

Low Carb Brownie

Prep time: 15 minutes | **Cook time:** 15 minutes | **Yield:** 8 servings

Ingredients:
- 1 cup coconut flour
- 1 tablespoon cocoa powder
- 1 tablespoon butter
- 1 teaspoon vanilla extract
- 1 teaspoon baking powder
- 1 teaspoon apple cider vinegar
- 1/3 cup coconut oil, melted
- 1 tablespoon Erythritol
- 1 cup water, for cooking

Method:
1. In the mixing bowl, mix up Erythritol, coconut oil, apple cider vinegar, baking powder, vanilla extract, butter, cocoa powder, and coconut flour.
2. Whisk the mixture until smooth and pour it into the baking pan. Flatten the surface of the batter.
3. Pour water and insert the steamer rack into the slow cooker.
4. Put the pan with brownie batter on the rack. Close and seal the lid.
5. Cook the brownie on manual mode (high pressure) for 15 minutes.
6. Then allow the natural pressure release for 5 minutes.
7. Cut the cooked brownies into the bars.

Nutritional info per serve: 155 calories, 2.1g protein, 10.6g carbohydrates, 12.6g fat, 5.2g fiber, 4mg cholesterol, 41mg sodium, 82mg potassium.

Berry Pudding

Yield: 4 servings | **Prep time:** 10 minutes | **Cook time:** 5 hours

Ingredients:
- ¼ cup strawberries, chopped
- 2 tablespoons Erythritol
- 2 cups of coconut milk
- 1 tablespoon almond flour
- 1 teaspoon vanilla extract

Method:
1. Mix coconut milk with almond flour and pour liquid into the slow cooker.
2. Add vanilla extract, Erythritol, and strawberries.
3. Close the lid and cook the pudding on low for 5 hours.
4. Carefully mix the dessert before serving.

Nutritional info per serve: 322 calories, 4.3g protein, 16.5g carbohydrates, 32.1g fat, 3.6g fiber, 0mg cholesterol, 21mg sodium, 331mg potassium.

Vanilla Flan

Prep time: 10 minutes | **Cook time:** 8 minutes | **Yield:** 4 servings

Ingredients:
- 4 egg whites
- 4 egg yolks
- ½ cup Erythritol
- 7 oz coconut cream, whipped
- 3 tablespoons water
- 1 tablespoon butter
- ½ teaspoon vanilla extract
- 1 cup water, for cooking

Method:
1. In the saucepan, heat Erythritol and butter. When the mixture is smooth, leave it in a warm place.
2. Meanwhile, mix up water, coconut cream, egg whites, and egg yolks. Whisk the mixture.
3. Pour the Erythritol mixture in the flan ramekins and then add heavy cream mixture over the sweet mixture.
4. Pour water and insert the steamer rack into the slow cooker.
5. Place the ramekins with flan on the rack. Close and seal the lid.
6. Cook the dessert on manual (high pressure) for 10 minutes. Then allow the natural pressure release for 10 minutes.
7. Cool the cooked flan for 25 minutes.

Nutritional info per serve: 212 calories, 7.5g protein, 3.7g carbohydrates, 19.3g fat, 1.1g fiber, 217mg cholesterol, 70mg sodium, 205mg potassium.

Lemon Cantaloupe Slices

Yield: 2 servings | **Prep time:** 10 minutes | **Cook time:** 3 hours

Ingredients:
- 2 cantaloupe slices
- 2 tablespoons lemon juice
- 1 tablespoon Erythritol
- 2 tablespoons butter

Method:
1. Sprinkle the cantaloupe slices with lemon juice and put them in the slow cooker.
2. Add butter and Erythritol.
3. Close the lid and cook the cantaloupe on low for 3 hours.

Nutritional info per serve: 129 calories, 0.8g protein, 13.5g carbohydrates, 11.8g fat, 0.7g fiber, 31mg cholesterol, 96mg sodium, 207mg potassium.

Vanilla Pie

Prep time: 20 minutes | **Cook time:** 35 minutes | **Yield:** 12 servings

Ingredients:

- 1 cup coconut cream
- 3 eggs, beaten
- 1 teaspoon vanilla extract
- ¼ cup Erythritol
- 1 cup coconut flour
- 1 tablespoon coconut oil, melted
- 1 cup water, for cooking

Method:

1. In the mixing bowl, mix up coconut flour, Erythritol, vanilla extract, eggs, and heavy cream.
2. Grease the baking pan with melted coconut oil.
3. Pour the coconut mixture into the baking pan.
4. Pour water and insert the steamer rack into the slow cooker.
5. Place the pie on the rack. Close and seal the lid.
6. Cook the pie on manual mode (high pressure) for 35 minutes.
7. Allow the natural pressure release for 10 minutes.

Nutritional info per serve: 112 calories, 3.2g protein, 12.9g carbohydrates, 8g fat, 4.4g fiber, 41mg cholesterol, 18mg sodium, 68mg potassium.

Vanilla Curd

Prep time: 5 minutes | **Cook time:** 5 minutes | **Yield:** 3 servings

Ingredients:

- 4 egg yolks, whisked
- 2 tablespoon coconut oil
- 1 tablespoon Erythritol
- ½ cup organic almond milk
- 1 teaspoon vanilla extract

Method:

1. Set the slow cooker in "Saute" mode and when the "Hot" is displayed – add coconut oil.
2. Melt the coconut oil but not boil it and add whisked egg yolks, almond milk, and vanilla extract.
3. Add Erythritol. Whisk the mixture.
4. Cook the meal on "Low" for 6 hours.

Nutritional info per serve: 246 calories, 4.5g protein, 8.2g carbohydrates, 24.6g fat, 0.9g fiber, 280mg cholesterol, 17mg sodium, 132mg potassium.

Custard

Prep time: 10 minutes | **Cook time:** 7 minutes | **Yield:** 4 servings

Ingredients:

- 6 eggs, beaten
- 1 cup coconut cream
- 1 teaspoon vanilla extract
- ¼ teaspoon ground nutmeg
- 2 tablespoons Erythritol
- 1 tablespoon coconut flour
- 1 cup water, for cooking

Method:

1. Whisk the eggs and Erythritol until smooth.
2. Then add coconut cream, vanilla extract, ground nutmeg, and coconut flour.
3. Whisk the mixture well again.
4. Then pour it in the custard ramekins and cover with foil.
5. Pour water and insert the steamer rack into the slow cooker.
6. Place the ramekins with custard on the rack. Close and seal the lid.
7. Cook the meal on manual (high pressure) for 7 minutes. Make a quick pressure release.

Nutritional info per serve: 244 calories, 9.9g protein, 12.8g carbohydrates, 21.1g fat, 2.1g fiber, 246mg cholesterol, 102mg sodium, 248mg potassium.

Dump Cake

Yield: 8 servings | **Prep time:** 15 minutes | **Cook time:** 5 hours

Ingredients:

- 1 keto cupcake mix
- 1 teaspoon vanilla extract
- ½ teaspoon ground nutmeg
- 1 tablespoon coconut
- oil, melted
- 2 eggs, beaten
- 1 teaspoon lemon zest, grated
- ½ cup coconut milk
- 4 pecans, chopped

Method:

1. In the bowl mix all ingredients except pecans.
2. Then line the slow cooker with baking paper and pour the dough inside.
3. Flatten the batter and top with pecans.
4. Close the lid and cook the dump cake for 5 hours on Low.
5. Cook the cooked cake well before serving.

Nutritional info per serve: 116 calories, 2.5g protein, 2.1g carbohydrates, 11.4g fat, 1.1g fiber, 41mg cholesterol, 18mg sodium, 85mg potassium

Lava Cake

Prep time: 15 minutes | **Cook time:** 18 minutes | **Yield:** 4 servings

Ingredients:

- 1 teaspoon baking powder
- 1 tablespoon cocoa powder
- 1 cup coconut cream
- 1/3 cup coconut flour
- 1 tablespoon almond flour
- 2 teaspoons Erythritol
- 1 tablespoon coconut oil, melted
- 1 cup water, for cooking

Method:

1. Whisk together baking powder, cocoa powder, coconut cream, coconut flour, almond flour, Erythritol, and coconut oil.
2. Then pour the chocolate mixture into the baking cups.
3. Pour water into the slow cooker. Insert the steamer rack.
4. Place the cups with cake mixture on the rack. Close and seal the lid.
5. Cook the lava cakes on manual (high pressure) for 4 minutes. Allow the natural pressure release for 5 minutes.

Nutritional info per serve: 222 calories, 3.3g protein, 14.2g carbohydrates, 19.7g fat, 5.9g fiber, 0mg cholesterol, 11mg sodium, 318mg potassium.

Zest Curd

Yield: 6 servings | **Prep time:** 15 minutes | **Cook time:** 7 hours

Ingredients:

- 1 cup coconut milk
- 1 tablespoon orange zest, grated
- 4 egg yolks
- 1/5 cup Erythritol
- 1 tablespoon almond flour
- 1 teaspoon vanilla extract

Method:

1. Whisk the egg yolks with Erythritol until you get a lemon color mixture.
2. Then add coconut milk, vanilla extract, almond flour, and orange zest. Whisk the mixture until smooth.
3. Pour the liquid into the slow cooker and close the lid.
4. Cook the curd on low for 7 hours. Stir the curd every 1 hour.

Nutritional info per serve: 158 calories, 3.7g protein, 4g carbohydrates, 14.9g fat, 1.5g fiber, 140mg cholesterol, 13mg sodium, 121mg potassium.

Cinnamon Roll

Prep time: 15 minutes | **Cook time:** 20 minutes | **Yield:** 4 servings

Ingredients:

- 1 tablespoon ground cinnamon
- 1 tablespoon coconut oil, softened
- 2 tablespoons almond butter
- 1 tablespoon
- Erythritol
- ½ cup almond flour
- ½ teaspoon baking powder
- 1 cup water, for cooking

Method:

1. In the mixing bowl, mix up almond butter, almond flour, and baking powder. Knead the dough.
2. Then roll it up and grease it with coconut oil.
3. Then sprinkle the dough with Erythritol and ground cinnamon.
4. Roll the dough into a log and cut on buns.
5. Pour water into the slow cooker and insert the steamer rack.
6. Put the cinnamon rolls (buns) in the baking pan and transfer them to the rack.
7. Close and seal the lid.
8. Cook the dessert on manual mode (high pressure) for 20 minutes. Make a quick pressure release.

Nutritional info per serve: 103 calories, 2.5g protein, 7.7g carbohydrates, 9.7g fat, 2.1g fiber, 0mg cholesterol, 2mg sodium, 131mg potassium.

Strawberries Bake

Yield: 4 serving | **Prep time:** 10 minutes | **Cook time:** 4 hours

Ingredients:

- 1 cup strawberries, chopped
- 1 tablespoon Erythritol
- 1 teaspoon lemon juice
- ½ teaspoon ground cinnamon

Method:

1. Put all ingredients in the slow cooker and stir well.
2. Close the lid and cook the meal on Low for 4 hours.
3. Carefully stir the cooked dessert and transfer it into the serving bowls.

Nutritional info per serve: 13 calories, 0.3g protein, 6.8g carbohydrates, 0.1g fat, 0.9g fiber, 0mg cholesterol, 1mg sodium, 58mg potassium.

Peanut Bars

Prep time: 25 minutes | **Cook time:** 12 minutes | **Yield:** 6 servings

Ingredients:

- 2 tablespoons coconut oil
- 2 oz peanuts, chopped
- 2 tablespoons Erythritol
- ½ teaspoon baking powder
- 4 tablespoons coconut flour
- 1 tablespoon almond butter, softened
- 1 teaspoon of cocoa powder
- 1 cup water, for cooking

Method:

1. Make the pie crust: knead the dough from almond butter, coconut flour, and baking powder.
2. Then put the dough in the pie mold and flatten it.
3. Pour water and insert the rack into the slow cooker.
4. Put the pie crust in the slow cooker. Close and seal the lid.
5. Cook it on manual mode (high pressure) for 12 minutes. Make a quick pressure release.
6. Meanwhile, mix up peanuts, coconut oil, Erythritol, and cocoa powder. Melt the mixture.
7. When the pie crust is cooked, pour the peanut mixture over it and cool it.

Nutritional info per serve: 130 calories, 3.7g protein, 10.7g carbohydrates, 11.2g fat, 3.2g fiber, 0mg cholesterol, 2mg sodium, 137mg potassium.

Vanilla Hot Drink

Prep time: 2 minutes | **Cook time:** 7 minutes | **Yield:** 2 servings

Ingredients:

- 1 cup coconut milk
- 1 teaspoon coconut oil
- 1 teaspoon vanilla
- extract
- 1 teaspoon erythritol
- 1 tablespoon cocoa powder

Method:

1. Transfer all the ingredients into the slow cooker bowl.
2. Set the "Saute" and start to cook the hot chocolate.
3. Saute the hot chocolate until it starts to boil. (around 10 minutes).

Nutritional info per serve: 308 calories, 3.2g protein, 10.9g carbohydrates, 31.2g fat, 3.4g fiber, 0mg cholesterol, 19mg sodium, 386mg potassium.

Cocoa Cookie

Prep time: 15 minutes | **Cook time:** 25 minutes | **Yield:** 4 servings

Ingredients:

- ½ cup almond flour
- 3 tablespoons cream cheese
- 1 teaspoon of cocoa powder
- 1 tablespoon Erythritol
- ¼ teaspoon baking
- powder
- 1 teaspoon apple cider vinegar
- 1 tablespoon coconut oil
- 1 cup water, for cooking

Method:

1. Make the dough: mix up almond flour, cream cheese, cocoa powder, Erythritol, baking powder, apple cider vinegar, and coconut oil. Knead the dough,
2. Then transfer the dough to the baking pan and flatten it in the shape of a cookie.
3. Pour water and insert the steamer rack into the slow cooker.
4. Put the pan with a cookie in the slow cooker. Close and seal the lid.
5. Cook the cookie on manual (high pressure) for 25 minutes. Make a quick pressure release. Cool the cookie well.

Nutritional info per serve: 77 calories, 1.4 g protein, 5.1g carbohydrates, 7.8g fat, 0.5g fiber, 8mg cholesterol, 24mg sodium, 52mg potassium.

Pecan Pralines

Prep time: 15 minutes | **Cook time:** 7 minutes | **Yield:** 4 servings

Ingredients:

- 4 pecans
- 4 teaspoons coconut oil
- 1 teaspoon of cocoa powder
- 1 teaspoon Erythritol

Method:

1. Heat the slow cooker on saute mode.
2. Then add coconut oil and cocoa powder. Saute the mixture until it is smooth and homogenous.
3. Meanwhile, line the tray with baking paper.
4. Put the pecans on the baking paper.
5. Pour the hot coconut oil mixture over the pecans. Refrigerate the pralines for 10-15 minutes.

Nutritional info per serve: 138 calories, 1.6g protein, 3.5g carbohydrates, 14.6g fat, 1.6g fiber, 0mg cholesterol, 0mg sodium, 69mg potassium.

Red Velvet Muffins

Prep time: 10 minutes | **Cook time:** 15 minutes | **Yield:** 2 servings

Ingredients:

- ¼ teaspoon keto red food coloring
- 2 teaspoons coconut oil
- ¼ teaspoon baking powder
- 1 teaspoon apple cider vinegar
- 4 tablespoons almond flour
- 1 teaspoon vanilla extract
- 3 tablespoons coconut cream
- 1 cup water, for cooking

Method:

1. In the mixing bowl, mix up red food coloring, coconut oil, baking powder, apple cider vinegar, almond flour, vanilla extract, and coconut cream.
2. Stir the mixture until it is smooth.
3. After this, pour the mixture into the muffin molds.
4. Pour water and insert the steamer rack into the slow cooker.
5. Place the muffin molds on the rack. Close and seal the lid.
6. Cook the muffins on manual (high pressure) for 15 minutes. Make a quick pressure release.

Nutritional info per serve: 182 calories, 3.5g protein, 4.8g carbohydrates, 16.5g fat, 2g fiber, 0mg cholesterol, 9mg sodium, 128mg potassium.

Pumpkin Spices Balls

Yield: 4 serving | **Prep time:** 15 minutes | **Cook time:** 2 hours

Ingredients:

- ½ cup butternut squash puree
- ¼ cup of Erythritol
- 4 tablespoons coconut flour
- 1 teaspoon olive oil

Method:

1. Mix butternut squash puree with Erythritol
2. Then add coconut flour and knead the soft dough.
3. Make the balls from the squash mixture.
4. After this, brush the slow cooker bottom with olive oil.
5. Put the pumpkin balls in the slow cooker in one layer and close the lid.
6. Cook the squash balls on High for 2 hours.

Nutritional info per serve: 80 calories, 2.2g protein, 8.9g carbohydrates, 3.2g fat, 5.8g fiber, 0mg cholesterol, 31mg sodium, 73mg potassium.

Lime Mugs

Prep time: 15 minutes | **Cook time:** 15 minutes | **Yield:** 2 servings

Ingredients:

- ½ cup of organic almond milk
- ½ teaspoon lime zest, grated
- 1/3 teaspoon baking powder
- 4 tablespoons
- coconut flour
- 1 egg yolk
- 1 tablespoon Erythritol
- 1 cup water (for slow cooker)

Method:

1. Whisk the almond milk gently and add lime zest.
2. Add baking powder and coconut flour.
3. After this, whisk the egg and add it to the coconut mixture. Add Erythritol.
4. Whisk the mixture until smooth and pour it into the mugs.
5. Cover the top of the mugs with the foil and make the small holes with the help of the toothpick.
6. Pour water into the slow cooker and insert the steamer rack.
7. Seal the lid and set the "steam" mode.
8. Cook the cakes on "steam" mode for 13 minutes + quick pressure release.
9. Chill the cakes for 5 minutes and discard the foil.

Nutritional info per serve: 226 calories, 4.7g protein, 12.6g carbohydrates, 18.1g fat, 7.4g fiber, 105mg cholesterol, 14mg sodium, 252mg potassium.

Mint Lava Cake

Yield: 6 servings | **Prep time:** 15 minutes | **Cook time:** 1 hour

Ingredients:

- 1 cup keto fudge cake mix
- 1 teaspoon dried mint
- 4 tablespoons avocado oil
- 2 eggs, beaten

Method:

1. Mix cake mix with dried mint, avocado oil, and eggs.
2. When the mixture is smooth, pour it into the ramekins and place it in the slow cooker.
3. Cook the lava cakes on High for 1 hour.

Nutritional info per serve: 34 calories, 2g protein, 0.7g carbohydrates, 2.7g fat, 0.4g fiber, 55mg cholesterol, 21mg sodium, 51mg potassium.

Spiced Pudding

Prep time: 10 minutes | **Cook time:** 30 minutes | **Yield:** 2 servings

Ingredients:
- 1 egg, beaten
- ¼ cup coconut cream
- 1 tablespoon Erythritol
- ¼ teaspoon pumpkin
- pie spices
- 1 teaspoon butter
- 1 cup of water (for slow cooker)

Method:
1. Whisk the egg and mix it up with coconut cream.
2. Add Erythritol and pumpkin pie spices. Stir the mixture.
3. Grease the cake pan with butter and transfer the pudding mixture inside.
4. Pour 1 cup of water into the slow cooker.
5. Put the pudding on the steamer rack in the slow cooker.
6. Cover the pudding with foil and secure edges.
7. Put the "Manual" mode (High pressure) for 20 minutes.
8. Make the natural pressure release for 10 minutes.
9. Chill the pudding for 10 hours before serving.

Nutritional info per serve: 118 calories, 3.5g protein, 9.5g carbohydrates, 11.3g fat, 0.7g fiber, 87mg cholesterol, 49mg sodium, 110mg potassium.

Blueberry Tapioca Pudding

Yield: 4 servings | **Prep time:** 10 minutes | **Cook time:** 3 hours

Ingredients:
- 4 teaspoons keto blueberry jam, sugar-free
- 4 tablespoons
- tapioca
- 2 cups of coconut milk

Method:
1. Mix tapioca with coconut milk and pour it into the slow cooker.
2. Close the lid and cook the liquid on low for 3 hours.
3. Then put the blueberry jam in 4 ramekins.
4. Cool the cooked tapioca pudding until warm and pour over the jam.

Nutritional info per serve: 112 calories, 4.1g protein, 7.3g carbohydrates, 2.5g fat, 0.1g fiber, 10mg cholesterol, 58mg sodium, 71mg potassium

Coconut Balls

Prep time: 5 minutes | **Cook time:** 8 minutes | **Yield:** 2 servings

Ingredients:
- 2 tablespoon coconut shred
- 1 egg, whisked
- 2 tablespoons coconut flour
- ¾ teaspoon vanilla
- extract
- 1 teaspoon Erythritol
- 1 tablespoon coconut oil
- 1 cup of water (for slow cooker)

Method:
1. Combine the whisked egg, coconut flour, coconut shred, and vanilla extract. Add coconut oil.
2. Add baking powder and Erythritol.
3. Make the balls from the coconut flour mixture.
4. Pour 1 cup of water into the slow cooker.
5. Insert the steamer rack inside and place the ramekin on it. Add coconut balls.
6. Close and lock the slow cooker lid.
7. Set the "Manual" mode for 8 minutes – high pressure. QPR
8. Chill the dessert for 5-10 minutes or until they are warm.

Nutritional info per serve: 175 calories, 3.8g protein, 9.9g carbohydrates, 14.7g fat, 4g fiber, 82mg cholesterol, 33mg sodium, 32mg potassium.

Caramel Pie

Yield: 6 servings | **Prep time:** 15 minutes | **Cook time:** 2 hours

Ingredients:
- 1 cup keto vanilla cake mix
- 4 eggs, beaten
- 1 teaspoon butter, melted
- 4 keto caramels, crushed

Method:
1. Mix vanilla cake mix with eggs and butter.
2. Pour the liquid into the slow cooker and sprinkle it with crushed candies.
3. Close the lid and cook the pie on high for 2 hours.
4. Then cool it and remove it from the slow cooker.
5. Cut the pie into 6 servings.

Nutritional info per serve: 48 calories, 3.7g protein, 0.2g carbohydrates, 3.6g fat, 0g fiber, 111mg cholesterol, 46mg sodium, 39mg potassium.

Turnip Cake Cups

Prep time: 15 minutes | **Cook time:** 10 minutes | **Yield:** 2 servings

Ingredients:

- 1 egg
- 1 tablespoon coconut oil
- 1 teaspoon Erythritol
- ¾ teaspoon vanilla extract
- ½ cup turnip, chopped
- 1 tablespoon macadamia nuts,
- crushed
- ¾ 2 tablespoons almond flour
- ¾ teaspoon ground cinnamon
- ¾ teaspoon baking powder
- 1 cup of water (for slow cooker)

Method:

1. Crack the egg in the mixing bowl and whisk it well with the help of the hand whisker.
2. Add Erythritol, vanilla extract, almond flour, ground cinnamon, and baking powder.
3. Stir well until smooth.
4. Then add macadamia nuts and turnip.
5. Mix up the batter with the help of the spoon until homogenous.
6. Pour the batter into the non-stick cake molds.
7. Then pour 1 cup of water into the slow cooker. Insert the steamer rack.
8. Transfer the cakes to the rack and close the slow cooker lid.
9. Seal the lid and set the "Manual" mode (High pressure) for 10 minutes. (QPR).
10. Chill the cakes for 10-15 minutes

Nutritional info per serve: 138 calories, 3.4g protein, 7.1g carbohydrates, 12.2g fat, 1.5g fiber, 82mg cholesterol, 55mg sodium, 303mg potassium.

Mint Brownies

Prep time: 20 minutes | **Cook time:** 10 minutes | **Yield:** 4 servings

Ingredients:

- 1 tablespoon cocoa powder
- 1 tablespoon Erythritol
- 2 egg yolks, whisked
- ¼ cup of organic almond milk
- 1 teaspoon coconut
- oil
- 1 teaspoon dried mint
- 3 tablespoons coconut flour
- 1 cup of water (for slow cooker)

Method:

1. Pour almond milk into the slow cooker bowl and start to cook it on "saute" mode.
2. Add cocoa powder.
3. After this, add coconut oil.
4. When the mixture is smooth – start to add whisked egg yolks gradually. Add coconut flour.
5. Whisk the mixture without stopping.
6. Add Erythritol and mint. Whisk it all the time. Then flatten it.
7. Cook the dessert on "manual" mode for 10 minutes (QPR for 5 minutes).
8. Cut the dessert into bars.

Nutritional info per serve: 97 calories, 2.7g protein, 9.4g carbohydrates, 7.7g fat, 3g fiber, 105mg cholesterol, 7mg sodium, 85mg potassium.

Avocado Bread

Prep time: 5 minutes | **Cook time:** 3 minutes | **Yield:** 4 servings

Ingredients:

- 1 avocado, mashed
- ½ teaspoon baking powder
- ¼ teaspoon apple cider vinegar
- 1 teaspoon vanilla extract
- 1 tablespoon swerve
- 1 egg, whisked
- ¼ cup coconut cream
- ½ cup almond flour
- 1 cup water (for slow cooker)

Method:

1. Combine the baking powder, apple cider vinegar, vanilla extract, swerve, and whisked egg.
2. Add coconut cream and almond flour.
3. Add mashed avocado.
4. Mix up the mixture until you get the homogenous texture.
5. Transfer the dough into the non-stick cake mold and flatten gently with the help of the spatula.
6. Wrap the mold in the aluminum foil.
7. Pour water into the slow cooker and insert the steamer rack. Place the mold on the rack and close the lid.
8. Cook the bread on the "Steam" mode for 20 minutes. Use the quick pressure release.
9. Chill the bread and remove it from the cake mold.

Nutritional info per serve: 242 calories, 5.7g protein, 9.2g carbohydrates, 21.1g fat, 5.2g fiber, 41mg cholesterol, 26mg sodium, 363mg potassium.

Nutmeg and Cinnamon Cake

Prep time: 15 minutes | **Cook time:** 10 minutes | **Yield:** 4 servings

Ingredients:

- 1 teaspoon ground nutmeg
- ½ teaspoon ground cinnamon
- 1 egg, whisked
- 1/3 teaspoon baking powder
- ½ cup almond flour
- 1 tablespoon coconut oil
- ¼ cup of water
- 1 cup water (for slow cooker)

Method:

1. Stir together the whisked egg and water.
2. Add coconut oil, almond flour, baking powder, ground cinnamon, and ground nutmeg.
3. Stir the mixture together until smooth and homogenous.
4. Transfer the dough into the non-stick cake pan and flatten it well with the help of the fingertips.
5. Pour 1 cup of water into the slow cooker bowl and insert the trivet.
6. Put the cake pan on the trivet and cover it with foil.
7. Coo the cake on "Manual" mode (High pressure) for 10 minutes + NPR.

Nutritional info per serve: 133 calories, 4.4g protein, 3.8g carbohydrates, 11.3g fat, 1.8g fiber, 41mg cholesterol, 21mg sodium, 60mg potassium.

Spoon Cake

Yield: 10 servings | **Prep time:** 15 minutes | **Cook time:** 2.5 hours

Ingredients:

- 2 cups keto cake mix
- 1 cup coconut milk
- 2 eggs, beaten
- 1 tablespoon avocado oil

Method:

1. Mix coconut milk with keto cake mix and egg.
2. Then avocado oil and blend the mixture until smooth.
3. Then place the baking paper in the slow cooker.
4. Pour the cake mix batter into the slow cooker, flatten it gently, and close the lid.
5. Cook the cake on High for 2.5 hours.
6. Then transfer the cooked cake to the plate.
7. Leave the cake until it is warm and cut into servings.

Nutritional info per serve: 198 calories, 22.5g protein, 9.5g carbohydrates, 8.4g fat, 5.4g fiber, 33mg cholesterol, 168mg sodium, 79mg potassium.

Classic Keto Pie

Yield: 6 servings | **Prep time:** 15 minutes | **Cook time:** 2 hours

Ingredients:

- 1 cup rutabaga, peeled, chopped
- 1 cup almond flour
- 4 eggs, beaten
- ¼ cup of Erythritol
- 1 tablespoon coconut oil, melted
- 1 teaspoon vanilla extract

Method:

1. Blend Erythritol with eggs for 2-3 minutes.
2. Then add coconut flour, coconut oil, vanilla extract, and mix until smooth.
3. Add rutabaga and carefully stir the mixture until homogenous.
4. After this, line the slow cooker bottom with baking paper and pour the dough inside.
5. Cook the pie on High for 2 hours on High.

Cook the cooked pie well.

Nutritional info per serve: 99 calories, 5g protein, 13.2g carbohydrates, 7.6g fat, 1.1g fiber, 109mg cholesterol, 47mg sodium, 119mg potassium.

Chocolate Fudge Cake

Yield: 6 servings | **Prep time:** 20 minutes | **Cook time:** 2 hours

Ingredients:

- ¼ cup of Erythritol
- 1 cup coconut flour
- 1 tablespoon cocoa powder
- 1 teaspoon baking powder
- 2 oz dark chocolate, chopped, sugar-free, keto
- 1/3 cup coconut milk
- 1 tablespoon coconut oil, softened

Method:

1. Mix flour with Erythritol, cocoa powder, baking powder, and coconut milk.
2. Stir the mixture until smooth and place in the slow cooker. (use the baking paper to avoid burning).
3. Then cook the mixture on high for 2 hours.
4. Meanwhile, mix coconut oil and dark chocolate, and melt them in the microwave oven.
5. When the fudge is cooked, pour the chocolate mixture over it and leave it to cool for 10-15 minutes as a minimum.
6. Cut the cake into servings.

Nutritional info per serve: 184 calories, 3.9g protein, 12.6g carbohydrates, 11g fat, 7.6g fiber, 2mg cholesterol, 50mg sodium, 177mg potassium.

Ramekin Red Cakes

Prep time: 10 minutes | **Cook time:** 15 minutes | **Yield:** 2 servings

Ingredients:

- ¼ teaspoon keto red food coloring
- 2 teaspoons coconut oil
- ¼ teaspoon baking powder
- 1 teaspoon lemon juice
- 4 tablespoons coconut flour
- 3 tablespoons organic almond milk
- 1 cup water, for cooking

Method:

1. Mix up red food coloring, coconut oil, baking powder, lemon juice, and coconut flour.
2. Add almond milk.
3. Stir the mixture until it is smooth.
4. After this, pour the mixture into the non-sticky ramekins.
5. Pour water and insert the steamer rack into the slow cooker.
6. Place the ramekins on the rack. Cook the muffins on manual (high pressure) for 15 minutes + quick pressure release.

Nutritional info per serve: 96 calories, 0.7g protein, 2.4g carbohydrates, 10g fat, 1g fiber, 0mg cholesterol, 4mg sodium, 123mg potassium.

Red Muffins

Yield: 10 servings | **Prep time:** 15 minutes | **Cook time:** 2 hours

Ingredients:

- 1 cup zucchini, grated
- 2 eggs, beaten
- 3 tablespoons coconut oil, softened
- 2 tablespoons cream
- cheese
- 1 cup coconut flour
- ¼ cup coconut milk
- ¼ cup of Erythritol
- 1 teaspoon baking powder

Method:

1. In the bowl mix eggs, coconut oil, cream cheese, coconut flour, coconut milk, Erythritol, and baking powder.
2. Carefully stir the mixture until you get a smooth batter.
3. Then add zucchini and stir the mixture with the help of the spoon.
4. Pour the batter into the muffin molds (fill ½ part of every mold) and place it in the slow cooker.
5. Cook the muffins on high for 2 hours.

Nutritional info per serve: 127 calories, 3.9g protein, 14.3g carbohydrates, 9.1g fat, 5.1g fiber, 35mg cholesterol, 45mg sodium, 110mg potassium.

.

Pecan Pudding

Yield: 6 servings | **Prep time:** 10 minutes | **Cook time:** 1.5 hours

Ingredients:

- 3 cups of coconut milk
- 4 pecans, grinded
- 1 teaspoon vanilla extract
- 1 tablespoon butter
- 2 tablespoons almond flour
- 1 tablespoon Erythritol

Method:

1. Mix coconut milk with almond flour and Erythritol and pour in the slow cooker.
2. Add vanilla extract and butter.
3. Then add pecans and close the lid.
4. Cook the pudding on High for 1 hour.
5. Then carefully mix it and cook it for 30 minutes on high more.

Nutritional info per serve: 373 calories, 4.3g protein, 11.1g carbohydrates, 38.4g fat, 3.9g fiber, 5mg cholesterol, 32mg sodium, 356mg potassium.

Measurement Conversion Charts

Measurement

Cup	Ounces	Milliliters	Tablespoons
8 cups	64 oz	1895	128
6 cups	48 oz	1420	96
5 cups	40 oz	1180	80
4 cups	32 oz	960	64
2 cups	16 oz	480	32
1 cups	8 oz	240	16
3/4 cups	6 oz	177	12
2/3 cups	5 oz	158	11
1/2 cups	4 oz	118	8
3/8 cups	3 oz	90	6
1/3 cups	2.5 oz	79	5.5
1/4 cups	2 oz	59	4
1/8 cups	1 oz	30	3
1/16 cups	1/2 oz	15	1

Weight

Imperial	Metric
1/2 oz	15 g
1 oz	29 g
2 oz	57 g
3 oz	85 g
4 oz	113 g
5 oz	141 g
6 oz	170 g
8 oz	227 g
10 oz	283 g
12 oz	340 g
13 oz	369 g
14 oz	397 g
15 oz	425 g
1 lb	453 g

Temperature

Fahrenheit	Celsius
100 °F	37 °C
150 °F	65 °C
200 °F	93 °C
250 °F	121 °C
300 °F	150 °C
325 °F	160 °C
350 °F	180 °C
375 °F	190 °C
400 °F	200 °C
425 °F	220 °C
450 °F	230 °C
500 °F	260 °C
525 °F	274 °C
550 °F	288 °C

Recipe Index